Oxygen's Journey: Powering Cells

Oxygen's Journey: Powering Cells

Olsen

First Printing, 2024

Through thick and thin, you were there. At rue friend indeed

TABLE OF CONTENTS

CHAPTER 1

General Introduction

1.1 Introduction

Energy needed to fuel metabolism is typically obtained through the oxidation of nutrient molecules such as glucose, culminating in the production of ATP. Notably, there are two distinct pathways of energy transfer that are used to synthesize ATP, namely aerobic and anaerobic metabolism. Each process yields unique benefits and characteristics, which when used in tandem make the numerous functions of our cells possible.

Under oxygen-limiting conditions, anaerobic respiration is the principal means of cellular energy production. The anaerobic pathway creates lactate as a final product and is favoured under conditions where aerobic metabolism cannot fulfill the energetic requirements such as during intense exercise. Anaerobically, ATP can be produced far quicker from carbohydrates than it can aerobically. Despite this, anaerobic metabolism is not generally the primary energy generator as it is far less efficient than aerobic metabolism. To compare, a single molecule of glucose generates 2 ATP anaerobically while aerobic metabolism generates 38 ATP molecules. In contrast with anaerobic metabolism, aerobic metabolism occurs within the mitochondria via the Kreb's cycle. This process requires O_2 and culminates with the production of ATP, CO_2 and water. The constant consumption of O_2 means that the mitochondria behave as an O_2 sink, which must be continually supplied.

1.2 O_2 transport dynamics

O_2 movement relies on either diffusion and/or convection. The diffusive movement of a gas is driven by partial pressure (PO_2) gradients with its direction of net transfer leaning towards sites of lower PO_2 levels. Thus, for most organisms, O_2 uptake begins from the external environment (site of highest PO_2) and terminates at the mitochondrion (the site of lowest PO_2). As simple diffusion is a slow process when compared with the metabolic processes of an organism, it is considered the rate-limiting step for aerobic metabolism. The diffusion of O_2 is further impeded by various resistances such as the respiratory medium (e.g. O_2 diffuses 10,000 times slower in water than in air) and any physical barriers separating the PO_2 gradients (outer epithelium or other tissues). Ultimately, the rate at which diffusion occurs is dictated by the magnitude of the pressure gradient, the resistance of the media, resistance of any barriers and the temperature. This principal is illustrated mathematically by Fick's law of diffusion describing O_2 uptake ($\dot{M}O_2$):

$$\dot{M}O_2 = K*A*((\Delta PO_2)/D)$$

Where k is Krogh's diffusion coefficient, A is the area of the gas exchange surface, ΔPO_2 is the difference in partial pressure between blood and inspired water and D is the thickness of the water-to-blood diffusion barrier. Often, simple diffusion alone is too slow to sustain the metabolism of multicellular organisms and therefore convection processes (ventilation and perfusion) are required to facilitate $\dot{M}O_2$.

Convection transports O_2 by physical movement, either the flow of blood in the circulatory system or the flow of water by ventilation. Convection of these two respiratory media facilitate diffusion by maximizing PO_2 gradients at the sites of $\dot{M}O_2$. Thus, at the gill, PO_2 remains high due to the constant flushing of inspired water while at the tissues deoxygenated blood is replaced with oxygenated blood.

Smaller organisms (usually less than 1 mm in diameter) have a relatively high surface-to-volume ratio and thus can sustain $\dot{M}O_2$ by simple diffusion, which requires that the distance that O_2 must travel within the organism is small relative to the large surface area that O_2 can pass across. Such a scenario is not possible in larger organisms as surface-to-volume ratios decline with increasing body size. Body complexity and metabolic requirements of an organism may also affect the limiting size for which simple diffusion can satisfy O_2 uptake requirements.

1.3 The larval fish model

The study of larval fish is an important sub-discipline in the area of comparative physiology research (Burggren et al., 2009). Studying fish through early development provides general ichthyologic knowledge, which can be applied to aquaculture and fisheries management. Moreover, understanding the impacts of environmental stressors on larval fishes can provide crucial insight into the impacts of global change on fish populations worldwide. From a practical viewpoint, larval fish can provide an opportunity to utilize powerful techniques such as genetic manipulation and advanced optical measurement systems such as the one used throughout this book, the scanning micro-optrode technique (SMOT). In addition, the ease of care, high fecundity and short generation times significantly ease some constraints when dealing with other vertebrate models. For the reasons listed above, the zebrafish (*Danio rerio*) has become a particularly popular organism of study and as such, the larval zebrafish was selected as a model organism for this book.

1.4 Metabolic allocation

The study of a larval stage fish presents unique considerations especially with respect to metabolism. To begin, the mass-specific MR of larvae is considerably higher than in juveniles and adults (Rombough, 1988). The high metabolic rate is due to the high demand for energy to support rapid growth. It has been shown that roughly 80% of the energy content of the yolk of an early stage fish is dedicated towards growth (Rombough, 2011). This presents a unique challenge for species with cleidoic eggs (energy is not exchanged with the outside environment) because prior to exogenous feeding, energy supply is limited to the energy content of the yolk. The composition of the yolk sac can vary greatly depending on the species but regardless, it is a structure of high nutrient content provided mainly by proteins and to a lesser extent, lipids and carbohydrates (Kamler, 2008). Overall, freshwater (FW) fishes utilize lipid as the dominant fuel source (Finn and Fyhn, 2010). This energy supports an extremely fast growth rate of around 150% of body weight gain per day being recorded in some species of larval fish (Smith and Ottema, 2006). With such a high rate of growth, little energy is left for other activities [roughly 15% when accounting for metabolic waste (Rombough 2011)]. One study on newly hatched rainbow trout (*Oncorhynchus mykiss*) found that the larvae could not exceed an increase of 20% of the routine metabolic rate (Ninness et al. 2006). It has been suggested that larvae can utilize an additive model of energy allocation in which increased energetic costs can be met by an increased energy expenditure, however, due to the closed-system nature of early larvae energy stores, once energetic costs exceed a certain level, a compensatory partitioning must take place, which leads to the reduction of energy allocated to other functions (Rombough 2011).

For larval fish, energy conversion is largely by aerobic metabolism (Finn and Fyhn, 2010; Rombough, 1988). Larval fish have low glycogen reserves, low activities of glycolytic enzymes and low tissue lactate concentrations even under stressful conditions (Rombough, 2011).

1.5 The respiratory system

Larval zebrafish do not possess fully developed gills and thus until about 14 days post-fertilization (dpf), the principal site of $\dot{M}O_2$ is the skin (Rombough and Moroz, 1997). This is made possible by the high surface area to volume ratio in larval zebrafish at 4 dpf. In addition, the water-to-blood O_2 diffusion barrier is thin consisting of an epidermis of only two cell layers

(4 µm) at the time of hatching (Glover et al., 2013; Le Guellec et al., 2004). Other morphological adaptations favouring increased cutaneous O_2 uptake include expansive sub-cutaneous vascular networks coupled with specialized cutaneous structures such as an enlarged yolk sac, broad medial finfolds or enlarged pectoral fins, all of which significantly increase the gas exchange surface area (Feder and Burggren, 1985). Taken together, these features allow $\dot{M}O_2$ to be principally met through cutaneous O_2 uptake while the gills are developing (Rombough, 1988).

In zebrafish at 28°C, primordial gills are formed at 3 dpf (Jonz and Nurse, 2005). At this point, short processes have emerged from the gill arches, forming early gill filaments. In rainbow trout larvae, roughly 80% of their $\dot{M}O_2$ occurs via gas exchange at the skin (Rombough and Ure, 1991), a figure which remains steady up until 23-28 days post-hatch (Fu et al., 2010). Even as adults, fish may rely on cutaneous gas exchange for a portion of their O_2 supply with some estimates reaching as high as 30% (Feder and Burggren, 1985). Further, if the environmental O_2 availability remains high, the respiratory surface of the gills will be less developed (Shadrin and Ozernyuk, 2002).

1.6 The cardiovascular system

The circulatory system of the larval zebrafish develops quickly with the formation of major blood vessels such as the cardinal vein, the cardinal artery and the axial and trunk vasculature occurring at 19 hpf (Mably and Childs, 2010). The early development of the cardiovascular system suggests that it may play an important role in the distribution of $\dot{M}O_2$ throughout the body, as it does in later stages of development. Indeed, the study of Hughes et al. (2019) showed that internal convection in larval zebrafish plays a significant role in O_2 transfer at 4 dpf. By using SMOT, to measure regional epithelial O_2 flux (JO_2), it was demonstrated that the lack of internal convection reduced JO_2 at the head and trunk. Internal convention probably facilitates

$\dot{M}O_2$ by helping to maintain boundary layer diffusion gradients (Hughes et al. 2019) rather than by increasing the O_2 carrying (or delivery) capacity of the circulatory system. Indeed, it is known that the presence or absence of the O_2 carrying pigment, hemoglobin, within the circulating blood has little impact on the $\dot{M}O_2$ of larval zebrafish (Pelster and Burggren, 1996) under normoxic conditions.

1.7 The integumentary system

As the flow and mixing of water decrease rapidly as the water-skin interface is approached, an external boundary layer adjacent to the skin develops which can become an O_2-depleted region surrounding the fish. This layer of stagnant water has been shown to create a significant resistance to cutaneous O_2 uptake because the partial pressure of O_2 in the water at the skin-water interface drives the diffusion of O_2 across the epithelium (Wells and Pinder, 1996a). To some extent, as O_2 falls within the boundary layer, it is replenished by O_2 provided by the movement of water across the body of the larva. Notably, larval rainbow trout and potentially larval zebrafish have been shown to use their pectoral fins to ventilate the skin surface and refresh the boundary layer O_2 (Zimmer et al., 2020). Regardless, the PO_2 of the boundary will always be lower than in the bulk flowing water.

The skin of the larval zebrafish is a key exchange surface for respiratory gases but also for salts (principally Na^+ and Cl^- ions). Throughout the epithelium, specialized cells regulating most of the ionic and osmotic needs of the larvae can be found. The cells, termed ionocytes, are enriched with mitochondria, specialized transporters and channels that facilitate the uptake of Na^+ and Cl^-. The ionoregulatory mechanisms of ionocyes have been extensively studied and are described in-depth in a later chapter. The majority of the ionocytes are concentrated along the outside of the yolk sac. Notably, the surface of the yolk sac of larval fish is highly vascularized, with a large surface area and a thin epithelium which provides a morphological advantage when considering diffusion (Wells and Pinder, 1996b). Despite this, O_2 uptake measurements taken using respirometry (Rombough and Ure, 1991) or intravascular PO_2 measurements using microelectrodes (Rombough, 1992) suggest that in salmonids, the yolk sac is no more effective at O_2 uptake than the thicker and less vascularized skin of the trunk. Furthermore, by the partitioning of the gills, yolk sac and body surface of Atlantic salmon (*Salmo salar L.*) larvae using a multi-chambered respirometer, the yolk sac was found to be a less effective gas exchanger than the rest of the body (Wells and Pinder, 1996b). In contrast, using the more sensitive technique of SMOT to measure regional JO_2, 4 dpf zebrafish larvae had a higher JO_2 at the yolk sac than the trunk (Hughes et al., 2019).

1.8 Environmental fluctuations

Ultimately, the ability for the larval zebrafish to obtain O_2 from the surrounding water is dependent on the environmental conditions. To sense environmental O_2, zebrafish possess chemosensory cells referred to as neuroepithelial cells (NEC) (Dunel-Erb et al., 1982). NECs appear on the gill arches from 3 dpf and become innervated by 7 dpf (Jonz and Nurse, 2005). NECs are also found on the skin at 24 h post fertilization (hpf) and may be responsible for initiating hypoxic ventilatory response by 48 hpf (Coccimiglio and Jonz, 2012). After 3 dpf, the cutaneous NECs will begin to be replaced by a NEC population formed on the gill filaments (Jonz and Nurse, 2005).

Zebrafish are native to the southeast Himalayan region and can be found in small rivers, streams and pools of water that can become slow-moving or stagnant (Engeszer et al., 2007). These environments can restrict O_2 cycling and become hypoxic creating a challenge for zebrafish to obtain sufficient O_2 to maintain aerobic demands. Moreover, during the monsoon season, environments become flooded and the ionic composition of the water can change drastically and alter the ionoregulatory demands of the zebrafish. Therefore, the zebrafish can serve as a useful model for studying the effects of altered environmental conditions on the capacity for O_2 uptake especially at the larval stage when the reliance on O_2 diffusion across the epithelium facilitates the usage of SMOT to monitor epithelial O_2 flux of local tissues and cells.

1.9 Hypotheses and predictions

Adequate uptake of O_2 is essential for maintaining aerobic metabolism. This research utilizes the technologically advanced method of SMOT to study epithelial O_2 flux in cutaneous respiring larval zebrafish. The technique and the chosen organism complement each other well in allowing a unique glimpse into a specific corner of respiratory physiology. Few studies have examined regional differences in O_2 consumption, and even fewer have measured differences in $\dot{M}O_2$ of specific cell types.

The first data chapter (Chapter 2) begins by describing the regional pattern of O_2 uptake across the epithelium. The chapter then progresses to test the interactive effects of hypoxia exposure and hypoxia inducible factor (HIF) on the epithelial O_2 flux. It was hypothesized that pre-exposure to hypoxia would increase the O_2 diffusing capacity of the skin of larval zebrafish via HIF-mediated increases in vascularization.

Chapter 3 examines regional O_2 uptake at the near-cellular level. For this study, the cutaneous ionocytes at the water interface were chosen as the target for SMOT. Because ionocytes contain an abundance of mitochondria and ATP-dependent transporters (Guh et al., 2015), they are presumed to have a high demand for O_2. The goal of this chapter was to manipulate Na^+ uptake rates as a method for quantifying the metabolic costs of ion regulation from the near cellular perspective. It was hypothesized that an altered Na^+ uptake rate would directly affect the O_2 uptake of the ionocytes. Therefore, the prediction followed that an increase in Na^+ uptake requires more energy to sustain and thus leads to an increase O_2 consumption of the Na^+ transporting ionocytes.

Chapter 2

Does hypoxia-inducible factor 1α play a role in regulating cutaneous oxygen flux in larval zebrafish (*Danio rerio*)

2.1 INTRODUCTION

The integument of fish is an important site of respiratory gas exchange especially for early developmental stages when larvae face the challenge of sustaining aerobic metabolism while the gills are still under development. Through whole-body respirometry and estimations of cutaneous surface area, it was found that newly hatched chinook salmon (*Oncorhynchus tshawytscha*) larvae (Rombough and Ure, 1991) and Atlantic salmon (*Salmo salar*) larvae (Wells and Pinder, 1996b) obtain roughly 80% of their O_2 through cutaneous gas transfer. Moreover, using microelectrodes to measure PO_2 surrounding the epithelium of rainbow trout (*Oncorhynchus mykiss* larvae, it was determined that that 73% of O_2 was obtained by cutaneous uptake (Rombough, 1998). Indeed, cutaneous O_2 uptake remains the dominant gas exchange organ in rainbow trout until 23-28 days post-hatch with the gills taking over after this point (Fu et al., 2010). Even through adulthood, fish may rely on cutaneous gas exchange for 10-20% of their O_2 supply with some estimates reaching as much as 30% (Feder and Burggren, 1985).

Notably, for embryonic (pre-hatch) and larval (post-hatch) stages of fish the morphometry of the young body displays a geometrically high surface area-to-volume ratio. It has been reported that larvae have an excess O_2 exchange capacity owing to the vast surface area of epithelium that can be used for gas exchange in comparison to the larval metabolic rate (Rombough and Moroz, 1997). In addition, the larval cutaneous diffusion distance is only slightly longer than that of lamellar diffusion distances in juvenile and adult fish (Rombough, 1988). The epithelium of larval fish is two cell layers thick at the point of hatching (Glover et al., 2013; Le Guellec et al., 2004) and the epithelium thickness has been estimated to range from 1.7 to 15 μm in larval stage fishes (Jones et al., 1966; Lasker, 1962; Roberts et al., 1973). Furthermore, in some species of larval fish, the cutaneous blood flow is arranged in a countercurrent exchange pattern with the water flowing across the body (Liem, 1981). Partially deoxygenated blood is brought to the skin by the caudal and rectal vascular systems of larval tilapia and the vitelline circulation in salmonids which increases partial pressure gradients across the blood and the skin (Rombough, 1988). Moreover, in larval zebrafish, internal convection provided by the cardiovascular system (Hughes et al., 2019) and possibly fin movement (Zimmer et al., 2020) can aid in the maintenance of respiratory gas transfer across the epithelium. Altogether, under normal conditions, the skin serves as an effective gas exchange organ to maintain the aerobic metabolism of a larval stage fishes.

In nature, fluctuations in environmental conditions can place pressure on the capacity for cutaneous O_2 uptake to meet the metabolic demands of the larvae. Aquatic hypoxia can be encountered during the warmer months when inhabited pools of water are warmed leading to a lower O_2 capacitance or when water flow is restricted due to evaporation, forming stagnant, hypoxic pools (Engeszer et al., 2007). If O_2 supply to the cells is reduced, then normal developmental velocity cannot be sustained (Rombough, 1988), leading to reduced growth in larval zebrafish (Schwerte, 2003). This is clearly not favourable for the fitness of the organism and therefore, it would be beneficial to improve the capacity of the skin as a gas exchanger to increase O_2 uptake and attempt to maintain normal energy levels for the crucial steps of early development. Considering the principles of O_2 diffusion (see Chapter 1 – General Introduction) there are many ways in which the cutaneous surface can be improved as a gas exchanger.

The rate-limiting barrier for O_2 diffusion is the boundary layer that is formed next to the epithelial surface. Therefore, larvae can enhance O_2 uptake by disturbing the stagnant, boundary layers to re-aerate the water closest to the skin. When exposed to hypoxia, larvae respond with an increase in body movements (Spoor, 1977; Spoor, 1984) and the pectoral fins (Green et al.,

2011; Holeton, 1971; Jonz, 2005; Liem, 1981) which have shown to create water currents along the body of larval zebrafish and Atlantic salmon (Green et al., 2011; Peterson, 1975). Finally, through SMOT, it was shown that rainbow trout larvae utilize pectoral fin movements to dissipate PO_2 boundary layers which aids in maintaining O_2 uptake under hypoxic conditions (Zimmer et al., 2020).

Cutaneous O_2 uptake can also be improved by increasing the effective surface area for exchange. For example, larval lake trout (*Salvelinus naymaycush*) (Garside, 1959) and larval herring (*Coregonus artedii*) (Brooke and Colby, 1980) show increased vascularisation of the yolk sac when reared in hypoxia. Larval zebrafish at 6 dpf showed 22% higher vascularisation of the intersegmental blood vessels in addition to increased cardiac output, stroke volume and end-diastolic volume when reared under hypoxia (Yaqoob and Schwerte, 2010). In addition, 12 dpf hypoxia-exposed zebrafish displayed significantly elevated blood perfusion of the trunk muscle while gut perfusion was reduced by 50% (Schwerte, 2003). Similar changes to the cutaneous surface and increased perfusion have been observed in emmersed fish including mudskipper (*Periophthalmus magnuspinnatus*) and the amphibious mangrove rivulus (*Kryptolebias marmoratus)* (Cooper et al., 2012; Glover et al., 2013). After 10 days of aerial acclimation of *K. marmoratus*, there was a significant increase in cutaneous surface vasculature (Cooper et al., 2012). Furthermore, when exposed to air, the pearl blenny (*Entomacrodus nigricans*; (Graham et al., 1985)) and the black prickleback (*Xiphister atropurpureus*; (Daxboeck and Heming, 1982)) dilate the epidermal blood vessels to increase the capacity of cutaneous gas exchange.

Finally, efficiency of cutaneous O_2 transfer can be enhanced by minimizing the O_2 diffusion distance across the water-blood barrier. The adult fish gills display a considerable plasticity regarding structure to balance respiratory and osmoregulatory challenges through the remodelling of the thickness and the surface area of the gill (Gilmour and Perry, 2018; LeBlanc et al., 2010; Perry, 1998; Sollid and Nilsson, 2006; Sollid et al., 2003). A thickening of the lamellar epithelium has been shown to severely impact O_2 uptake in rainbow trout during hypoxia exposure (Bindon et al., 1994; Greco et al., 1996) and under extreme cases, can impact O_2 uptake in normoxia (Perry, 1998; Perry et al., 1996; Thomas et al., 1988). Thus, larval fish may reduce epithelium thickness when O_2 uptake is challenged to improve the efficiency of the skin as a gas exchange organ.

The transcription factor, hypoxia-inducible factor 1a (Hif-1α) plays a key role in maintaining O_2 homeostasis (Semenza, 2001). Under low O_2, Hif-1α accumulates within cells to enact several transcriptional changes. Hif-1α has been found to have impacts on metabolism, erythropoiesis, apoptosis, cell survival and proliferation (Semenza, 2003). Moreover, Hif-1α has also plays an essential role in facilitating angiogenesis (Gerri et al., 2017) and the hypoxic ventilatory response (Mandic et al., 2019) resulting in a reduction in the critical O_2 (P_{crit}) of zebrafish larvae previously exposed to hypoxia (Mandic et al., 2020; Robertson et al., 2014). Despite these findings, there is, yet, no direct evidence that increases in Hif-1α expression during hypoxia influences cutaneous PO_2 boundary layers and thus aids overall cutaneous O_2 uptake.

2.1.1 Hypotheses and predictions

The two main goals of this study were, first, to characterize the epithelium of the larval zebrafish as a gas exchange organ under normoxia and after a previous exposure to hypoxia and second, to evaluate the role of Hif-1α in managing larval cutaneous O_2 uptake. To achieve the first, a regional map of cutaneous JO_2 across the surface of 4 and 7 dpf larval zebrafish under normoxia. Next, whole-body O_2 consumption ($\dot{M}O_2$) and P_{crit} were measured along with trunk vascularity. It was hypothesized that if larvae were exposed to hypoxia, then the cutaneous gas exchange organ of the larvae would be affected. It was predicted that regional JO_2 and combined JO_2 determined by taking the sum of JO_2 across the larvae would by significantly higher in larvae pre-treated with hypoxic water. Based on previous literature it was predicted that $\dot{M}O_2$ under normoxia would remain unchanged, P_{crit} would decrease and trunk vascularity would increase with prior hypoxia exposure. These changes would highlight an increased hypoxia tolerance in the hypoxia-exposed larvae. Consequently, it was hypothesized that Hif-1α plays a major role in regulating the hypoxia-triggered increase in cutaneous O_2 uptake capacity. To test, I assessed whether a genetic knockout of both Hif-1α paralogues (Hif1aa$^{-/-}$ ab$^{-/-}$) would prevent the adaptive responses of larvae that were previously exposed to hypoxia. It was predicted that JO_2, $\dot{M}O_2$, P_{crit} and trunk vascularity in Hif1aa$^{-/-}$ ab$^{-/-}$ larvae would remain constant after hypoxia pre-exposure.

2.2 MATERIAL AND METHODS

2.2.1 Fish care and breeding

Wild-type (WT) zebrafish (*Danio rerio*) were housed at the University of Ottawa aquatic care facility. The Hif1aa$^{-/-}$ ab$^{-/-}$ and transgenic lines, generated via TALEN and CRISPR/Cas9 technologies (Gerri et al., 2017). Fish were maintained in plastic aquaria which were constantly supplied with aerated, dechloraminated City of Ottawa tap water at 28°C (referred to as "system water"; in mM: 0.25 Ca^{2+}, 0.78 Na^{+}, 0.4 Cl^{-}, 0.025 K^{+}, 0.15 Mg^{2+}; pH 7.6). Fish were kept on a 14 h light: 10 h dark photoperiod and fed until satiation with no. 1 crumble-Zeigler (Aquatic Habitats; Apoka, FL) once a day. Embryos were obtained through standard protocol (Westerfield, 2007) by breeding adult zebrafish in plastic 2 L breeding traps with a perforated insert. For breeding, 8 – 10 fish at a ratio of 2 females to 1 male were placed in breeding traps and left overnight. The following morning, embryos were collected using a fine mesh sieve and were placed in 50 mL petri dishes at a density of 30 embryos per dish containing different media, based on experimental protocols (see below), and held in an incubator set to 28.5°C. Media in the petri dishes was replaced daily until experimentation at 4 dpf. All experiments were conducted in compliance with the Canadian Council of Animal Care guidelines and after approval of the University of Ottawa Animal Care Committee (protocols BL-2118 and BL-1700).

2.2.2 Hypoxia exposure

Treatment groups designated as hypoxia-exposed were reared until 2 days post fertilisation (dpf) in normoxia (153 mmHg), after which, larvae were exposed to 6 h of hypoxia (40 mmHg) and then returned to normoxia until 4 or 7 dpf, for experimentation. The hypoxia exposure parameters were chosen as they have been shown to elicit the Hif-1α mediated blood vessel repair system (Gerri et al., 2017). All other treatment groups were reared in normoxia until 4 or 7 dpf. For the hypoxia exposure, 20 larvae of a single genotype were placed within a partially submerged cylindrical chamber, fitted with a mesh-covered bottom which allowed mixing of hypoxic water contained within a larger 30 l plastic tank. By mixing the appropriate quantities of air and N_2 within a water equilibration column, hypoxic water with a PO_2 of 40 mmHg was used to fill the plastic tank. A custom gas mixer fabricated at the University of Ottawa provided the gas mixtures and PO_2 and temperature of the water was monitored with a fiber optic O_2 and temperature meter (FireStingO_2, PyroScience, Aachen, Germany). After 6 h, larvae were removed from the cylindrical chambers and transferred to petri dishes filled with normoxic water and kept at 28.5°C until 4 or 7 dpf.

2.2.3 Regional SMOT measurements

The SMOT system consists of a fibre optic oxygen optrode (PreSens Precision Sensing GmbH, Regensburg, Germany) connected to a detector system and motion control unit developed by Applicable Electronics (Science Wares, Inc., Falmouth, MA, USA). Oxygen optrodes were constructed from fiber optic cables that were flame-pulled to a 40 μm tip and coated with Pt(II) meso-Tetra(pentafluorophenyl)porphyrin (Pt-TFPP; Frontier Scientific, Newark, DE, USA). The optrode was connected to the detector system that emits an excitation light through a blue LED ($\lambda = 400$ nm) that excites the Pt-TFPP coating and detects fluorescence emission. The fluorescent emission from Pt-TFPP is quenched in the presence of oxygen. The position of the optrode was manipulated using an Applicable Electronics CMC-4 (Applicable Electronics, New Haven, CT, USA) computer motion control unit and recordings were measured using ASET-LV4 software (Applicable Electronics). Larvae at 4 or 7 dpf were placed within a dish containing normoxic water and tricaine (0.2 g/L) buffered to pH 7.6. Arbitrary regions were designated across the surface of a larval zebrafish. The SMOT probe was placed in the center of each point along the larvae and JO_2 was measured five times with an excursion distance of 100 microns and a probe tip of 40 microns. Measurements started at the tail and progressed towards the head. A previous experiment (data not shown) revealed that starting at the tail or head did not impact JO_2. Using Microsoft Excel, a "heat map" of JO_2 was created using the grid overlay with green denoting the lowest JO_2 measurement and red indicating the highest.

2.2.4 Vascularisation

A double transgenic line Tg(fli1:EGFP)^{y1} Tg(gata1:dsRed) from Dr. Grosell's lab (Miami, Florida, USA) were utilized to determine vascularisation for each treatment. This line displayed vascular-specific expression of enhanced green fluorescent protein (EGFP) (Lawson and Weinstein, 2002) and fluorescing DsRed within red blood cells (Long et al., 1997). The double transgenic line was crossed with the Hif1aa$^{-/-}$ ab$^{-/-}$ line to visualize vascularisation of the knockout and wild-type genotypes.

At 2 dpf, larvae from the double transgenics and double transgenic x Hif1aa$^{-/-}$ ab$^{-/-}$ were either exposed to hypoxia at 40 mmHg for 6 h or maintained in normoxic water. At 4 and 7 dpf, larvae were anesthetized and placed on a concave microscope slide. Images were taken using a single photon, scanning confocal laser microscope (A1R^{+}, Nikon Instruments, Melville, NY, USA) with a 10x objective. Blood vessels were observed using a krypton–Argon laser at 480 nm and images were captured using step intervals of 3 µm.

Images were analyzed using Image-J 1.51 open source software (National Institutes of Health, Bethesda, MD, USA). The plugins Skeletonize (2D/3D) and Analyze Skeleton (2D/3D) were used to determine the number of vessel segments, end points, junctions, total vessel length and mean vessel length of the intersegmental blood vessels (ISVs) and the dorsal longitudinal anastomotic vessel (DLAV). A vascularisation index was calculated by multiplying the total vessel length by the number of junctions. The macro developed by Simms et al. (2017) was used to process images. First, images were cropped to include only the ISVs and the DLAV. Next, images were binarized, and the Fill Holes and Despeckle functions were applied. Finally, the image was skeletonized, and the Analyze Skeleton function was used.

2.2.5 Micro-respirometry

The system (Loligo Systems, Viborg, Denmark) consisted of a 24-well, glass microplate in which each chamber had a volume of 80 µL (well inner diameter d = 4.5 mm). Each well contained a non-invasive O_2 sensor spot, which was scanned by a 24-channel optical fluorescence O_2 microplate reader. The microplate was placed in a temperature-controlled (28.9

°C) water bath held on a shaker (continuous circular oscillations set to 30 RPM with a deviation of 25 mm) to prevent the formation of unstirred layers of water surrounding each larva. The sensors were calibrated using zero solution (20 g/L anhydrous Na_2SO_3) and air-saturated water. To ensure the contents of the microplate were sealed, PCR tape was placed over each well and then a silicone pad and a compression block were placed on top. Care was taken to remove air bubbles from the wells before recording PO_2. Following calibration, wells were rinsed thoroughly and larvae from each respective treatment were assigned randomly to wells (1 larva per well). PO_2 was recorded continuously for approximately 60 min.

O_2 consumption ($\dot{M}O_2$; pmol mg^{-1} h^{-1}) was calculated using the following equation:

$$\dot{M}O_2 = (\Delta PO_2 * \alpha O_2 * V)/m \quad (2)$$

where ΔPO_2 is the rate of change of PO_2 (mm Hg h^{-1}) within the chamber over time, αO_2 is the O_2 solubility constant (pmol L^{-1} $mmHg^{-1}$) in water at 30 °C (Boutilier et al., 1984), V is the volume (L) of the chamber and m is the average mass of the larva (mg). Wet mass was determined by placing 40 X 4 or 7 dpf larvae (anaesthetized by placing on ice) in a small, pre-weighed insert lined with a fine mesh, which was fixed atop a 50 mL falcon tube. To remove excess water, the bottom of the mesh was blotted with a tissue and then centrifuged at 400 rpm for 1 min. The fine mesh cup containing the larvae was then reweighed on an analytic balance to obtain the mass of the pool of 40 larvae (n = 1), which was used to estimate individual mass of the larva in the respirometer.

To calculate P_{crit}, the inflection point was determined from a plot of $\dot{M}O_2$ versus water PO_2 (binned to 6 min intervals) using a 'broken-stick' or segmented linear regression (Yeager and Ultsch, 1989) facilitated by REGRESS software (www.wfu. edu/~mudayja/software/o2.exe) for each trial.

2.2.6 Statistical analysis

All statistical analyses were performed using SigmaPlot (version 11.0; Systat Software, Chicago, IL, USA). Data are reported as means ± standard error of the mean (s.e.m.). Statistical significance of treatment effects was evaluated through two-way and one-way analysis of variance (ANOVA) followed by a Holm-Sidak *post-hoc* test. Statistical significance was accepted at $P \leq 0.05$. Specific details of statistical analyses are included in corresponding figure captions.

2.3 Results

2.3.1 Regional JO_2 maps

At 4 and 7 dpf there was a wide range of JO_2 along the cutaneous surface of the zebrafish larvae (Figs. 2.1 and 2.4) (n = 7-8). Across all maps, JO_2 was highest at the anterior end of the larva and decreased towards the middle and posterior ends (Figs. 2.2B and 2.5B) (two-way ANOVA; $p < 0.05$; n = 7-8). Within each region there was no difference in JO_2 for each treatment and genotype combination. There was no difference in combined JO_2 between WT and Hif1aa$^{-/-}$ab$^{-/-}$ larvae nor between normoxia- and hypoxia-exposed larvae at 4 dpf and 7 dpf (Figs. 2.2C and 2.5C).

2.3.2 Micro-respirometry

At 4 dpf, WT larvae (normoxia- and hypoxia-exposed) had a significantly higher $\dot{M}O2$ compared to the Hif1aa$^{-/-}$ab$^{-/-}$ larvae (Fig. 2.3A) (two-way ANOVA; $p < 0.05$; n = 29). At 7 dpf,

WT and Hif1aa$^{-/-}$ab$^{-/-}$ larvae pre-exposed for 6 h to hypoxia exhibited a significantly lower $\dot{M}O_2$ compared to larvae reared under normoxia (Fig. 2.6A) (two-way ANOVA; $p = 0.04$; $n = 6$-12). Measurements of P_{crit} at 4 dpf showed no statistically significant difference between either genotype or treatment (Fig. 2.3B) but there was a significant difference at 7 dpf with WT larvae showing a lower P_{crit} than Hif1aa$^{-/-}$ab$^{-/-}$ larvae (Fig. 2.6B) (two-way ANOVA; $p < 0.05$; $n = 9$-18).

2.3.3 Trunk vascularisation

At 4 and 7 dpf there was no difference in the vascularisation index between different genotypes and different treatments (Fig. 2.8) (two-way ANOVA; $p > 0.05$; $n = 4$-8). Similarly, there was no significant difference between the individual parameters of number of vessel junctions and total vessel length between the different treatments and genotypes. Additionally, all other parameters that were obtained are presented in table 1 for reference.

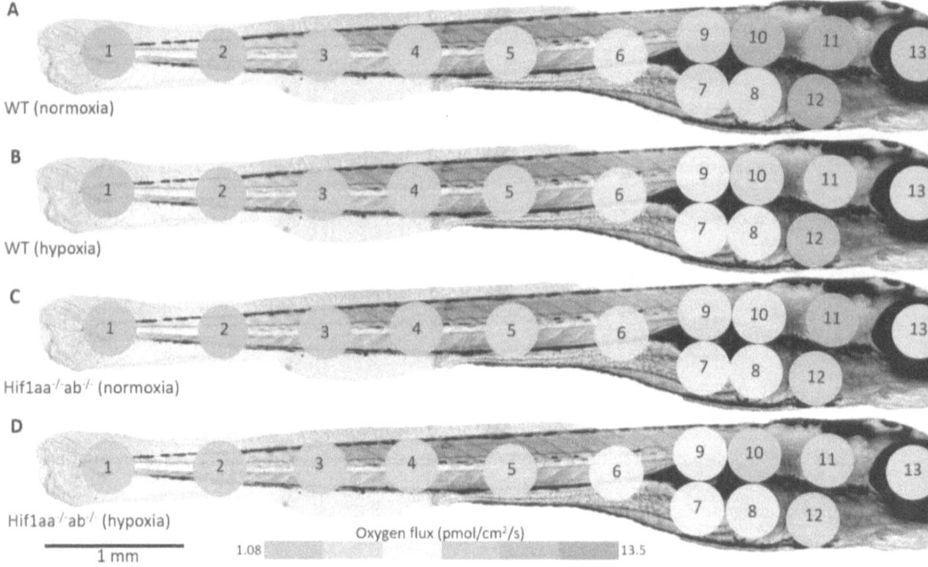

Figure 2.1. Oxygen flux (JO_2) measured across the surface of a 4 days post-fertilisation (dpf) wild-type and Hif1aa$^{-/-}$ab$^{-/-}$ larval zebrafish reared in normoxia (A-B) and 40 mmHg hypoxia for 6 h at 2 dpf (C-D). The lowest area of JO_2 was set as dark green and the highest JO_2 as dark red with all the colours in-between denoting intermediate values of JO_2. Each coloured circle was arbitrarily set and sized. JO_2 was measured in the middle of each circle. n = 7-8.

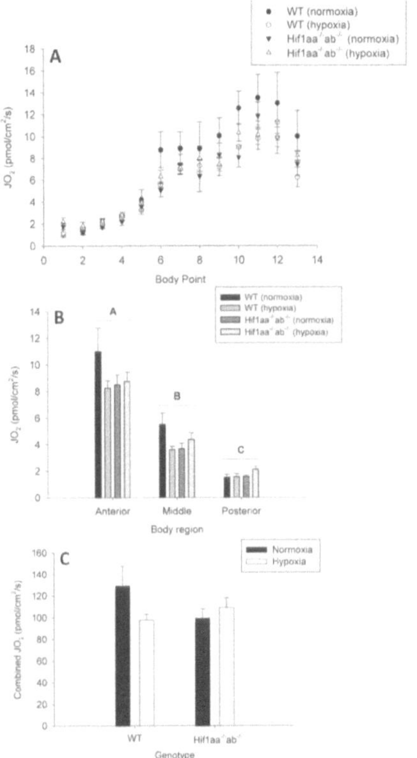

Figure 2.2. Cutaneous oxygen flux (JO_2) across the surface of 4 days post-fertilisation (dpf) wild-type and Hif1aa$^{-/-}$ab$^{-/-}$ larval zebrafish reared in normoxia or pre-exposed to 40 mmHg hypoxia for 6 h at 2 dpf. JO_2 was presented by body point (A), regionally (B) and as a combined, whole-body JO_2 (C). The regions were marked by separating the larvae into three equal lengths and averaging the JO_2 of each body point found within the region. With reference to Figure 2.1, the posterior includes points 1-3, middle 4-6 and anterior 7-13. The combined JO_2 was calculated by finding the sum of the JO_2 at each body point (A) for each treatment. Letters represent a

statistically significant difference between body region (two-way ANOVA; $p < 0.05$; n = 7-8). Data are presented as means ± SEM.

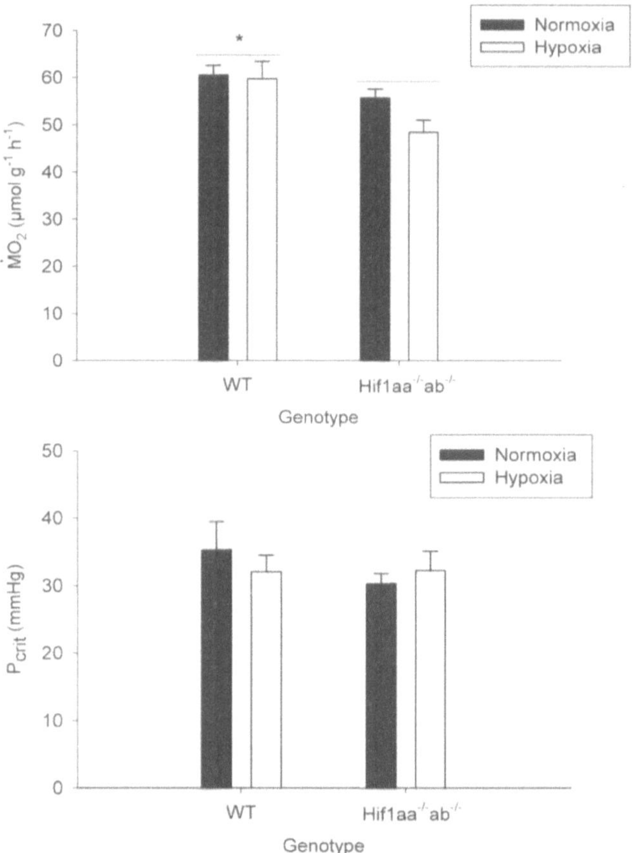

Figure 2.3. Whole-body O_2 consumption ($\dot{M}O_2$; A) and critical O_2 tension (P_{crit}; B) of 4 days post-fertilisation (dpf) wild-type and Hif1aa$^{-/-}$ab$^{-/-}$ larval zebrafish reared in normoxia or pre-exposed to 40 mmHg hypoxia for 6 h at 2 dpf. An asterisk denotes a significant difference between genotypes (two-way ANOVA; $p < 0.05$; n = 29). Data are presented as means ± SEM.

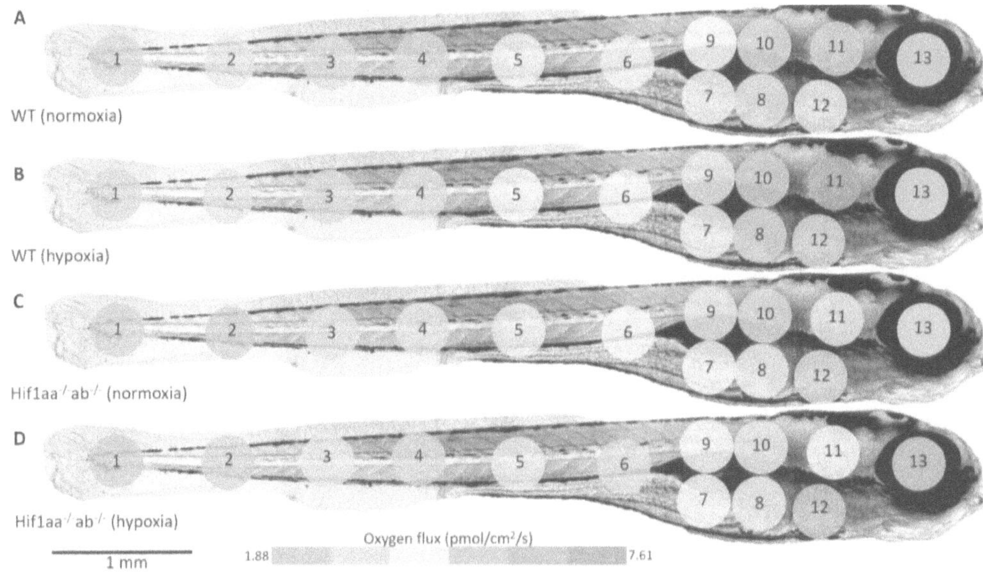

Figure 2.4. Oxygen flux (JO_2) measured across the surface of a 7 days post-fertilisation (dpf) wild-type and Hif1aa$^{-/-}$ab$^{-/-}$ larval zebrafish reared in normoxia (A-B) and 40 mmHg hypoxia for 6 h at 2 dpf (C-D). The lowest area of JO_2 was set as dark green and the highest JO_2 as dark red with all the colours in-between denoting intermediary values of JO_2. Each coloured circle was arbitrarily set and sized. JO_2 was measured in the middle of each circle. n = 4-6.

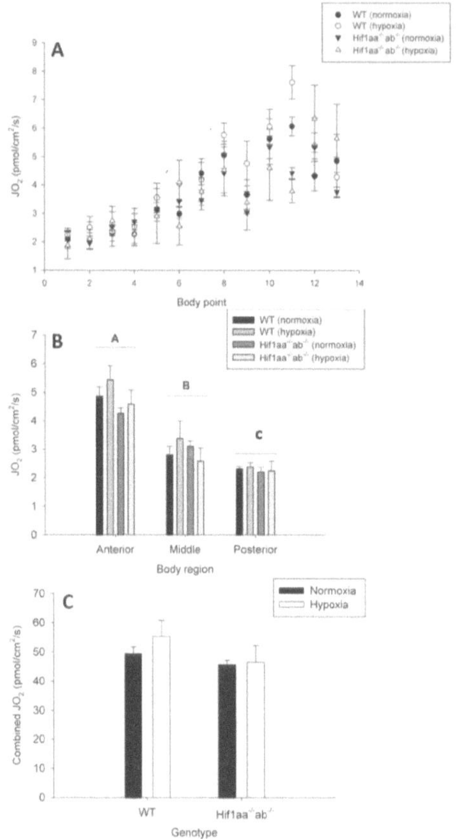

Figure 2.5. Cutaneous oxygen flux (JO_2) across the surface of 7 days post-fertilisation (dpf) wild-type and Hif1aa$^{-/-}$ab$^{-/-}$ larval zebrafish reared in normoxia or pre-exposed to 40 mmHg hypoxia for 6 h at 2 dpf. JO_2 was presented by body point (A), regionally (B) and as a combined, whole-body JO_2 (C). The regions were marked by separating the larvae into three equal lengths and averaging the JO_2 of each body point found within the region. With reference to Figure 2.4, the posterior includes points 1-3, middle 4-6 and anterior 7-13. The combined JO_2 was calculated by finding the sum of the JO_2 at each body point (A) for each treatment. Letters

represent a statistically significant difference between body region (two-way ANOVA; $p < 0.05$; $n = 4\text{-}6$). Data are presented as means ± SEM.

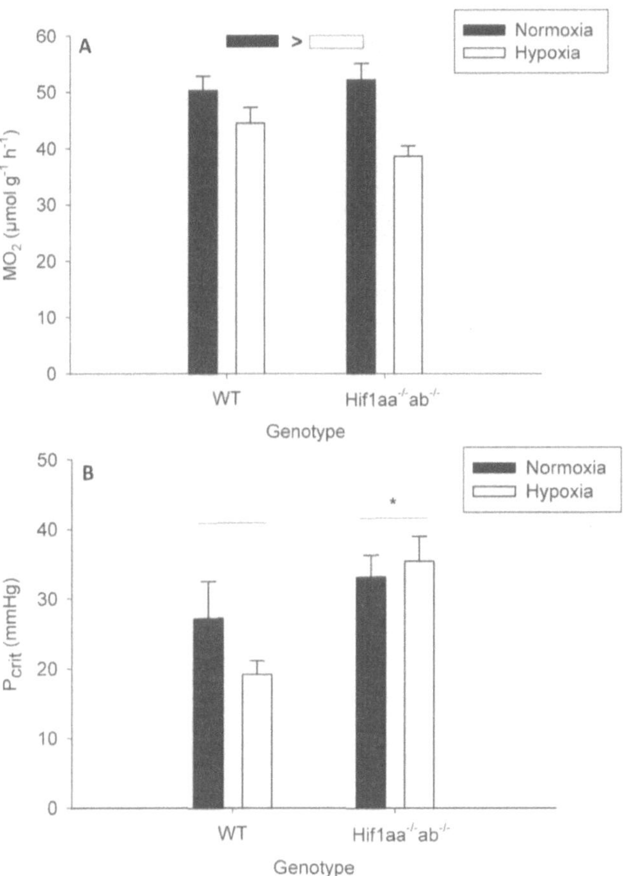

Figure 2.6. Whole-body O_2 consumption ($\dot{M}O_2$; A) and critical O_2 tension (P_{crit}; B) in wild-type and Hif1aa$^{-/-}$ab$^{-/-}$ 7 days post-fertilisation (dpf) larvae reared in normoxia and or pre-exposed to 40 mmHg hypoxia for 6 h at 2 dpf. An asterisk denotes a significant difference between genotypes (two-way ANOVA; $p < 0.05$; $n = 9\text{-}18$). Data are presented as means ± SEM.

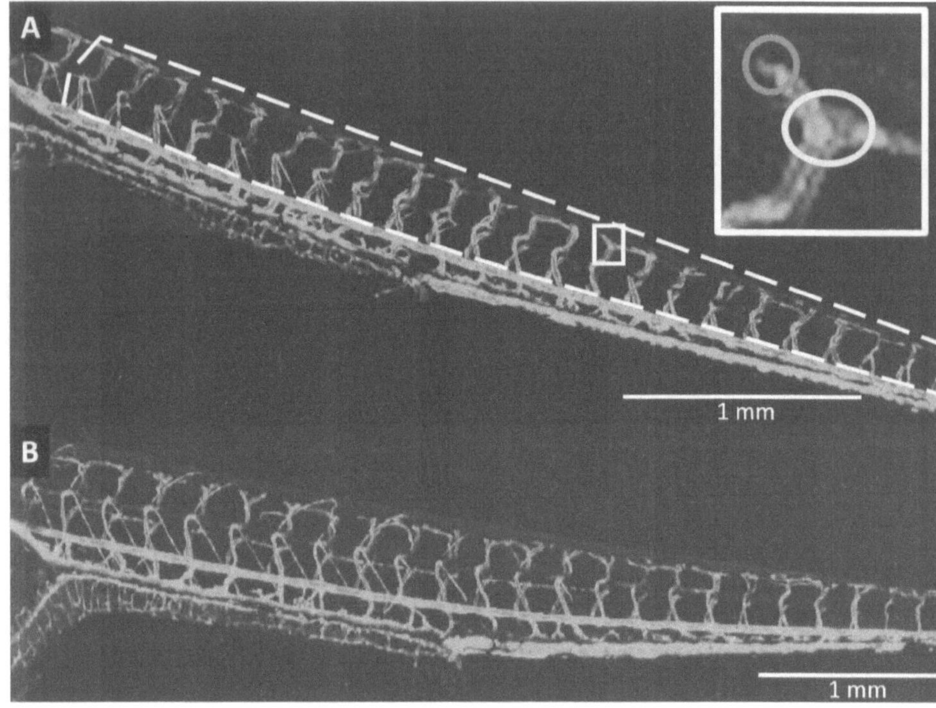

Figure 2.7. Representative images of 4 (A) and 7 (B) days post-fertilisation, (dpf) transgenic, fli;eGFP zebrafish larvae. The dotted white line denotes the region which was used to measure vascularity which comprises the intersegmental vessels and the dorsal longitudinal anastomotic vessel. The white box is a magnified portion of the trunk vasculature to illustrate an example of a vessel endpoint (red circle) and a junction (yellow circle).

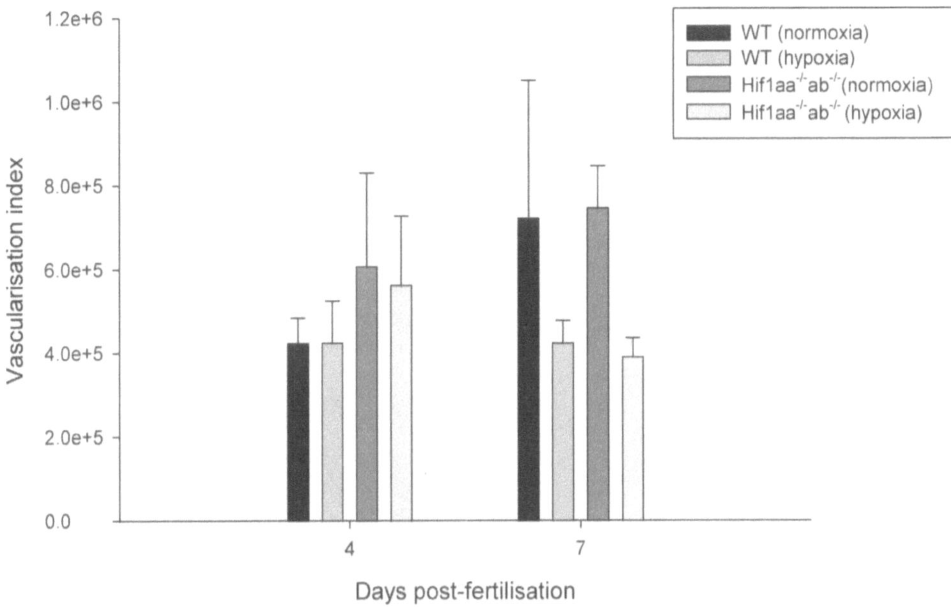

Figure 2.8. Analysis of the vascularity of the intersegmental vessels and the dorsal longitudinal anastomotic vessels of wild-type and Hif1aa$^{-/-}$ab$^{-/-}$ 4- and 7-days post-fertilisation (dpf) larvae reared in normoxia or pre-exposed to 40 mmHg hypoxia for 6 h at 2 dpf. To visualize blood vessels, fli;eGFP transgenic zebrafish were used. Vasculature was analysed using ImageJ to determine the vascularisation index. The index was calculated by multiplying the total vessel length (in pixels) by the number of vessel junctions. Data are presented as means ± SEM. (n = 8).

Table 2.1. Analysis of the vascularity of the intersegmental vessels and the dorsal longitudinal anastomotic vessel of wild-type and Hif1aa$^{-/-}$ab$^{-/-}$ 4- and 7-days post-fertilisation (dpf) larvae reared in normoxia and 40 mmHg hypoxia for 6 hours at 2 dpf. To visualize blood vessels, fli;eGFP transgenic zebrafish were used. Vasculature was analysed using ImageJ to determine the blood vessel parameters (Simms et al., 2017). Results were compiled using Microsoft Excel. Data are presented as means ± SEM. (n = 8).

		Blood vessel parameters				
Age (dpf)	Treatment	# of segments	# of junctions	# of endpoints	Total vessel length	Mean vessel length
4	WT	100±14	91±8	250±18	4284±465	12± 1
	WT (hypoxia)	109±21	93±11	307±46	4230±607	15±2
	Hif1aa$^{-/-}$ab$^{-/-}$	145±20	106±26	385±55	4844±973	14±1
	Hif1aa$^{-/-}$ab$^{-/-}$ (hypoxia)	94±18	112±15	298±50	4653±665	14±1
7	WT	128±11	111.1±20	356±31	5103±620	14.9±0.6
	WT (hypoxia)	120±16	80±12	317±35	3943±680	14±1.3
	Hif1aa$^{-/-}$ab$^{-/-}$	138±17	116±6	390±36	5688±372	15±0.3
	Hif1aa$^{-/-}$ab$^{-/-}$ (hypoxia)	146±9	96±7	383±22	4862±487	15±0.1

2.5 DISCUSSION

2.5.1 Spatial profile of JO_2

In Chapter 2, a detailed map of regional JO_2 was created across the epithelium of 4 and 7 dpf larval zebrafish. The maps reveal a diverse range of JO_2 across the skin. This finding concurs with PO_2 measurements across the epithelium of larval rainbow trout using microelectrodes (Rombough, 1992). The PO_2 measured at the skin-water interface by Rombough (1992) varied from 7% (around the yolk sac) to 36% (caudal fin) of the free-stream PO_2. The spatial pattern of O_2 sinks in larval rainbow trout match that of larval zebrafish with the lowest JO_2, measured at the caudal fin and the highest JO_2 around the heart and developing gills. Indeed, it appears that the yolk sac does not play the major role in O_2 uptake for larval fish as was previously thought (Rombough, 1988; Rombough and Moroz, 1997). Based on morphological considerations, the thin and well-vascularized integument of the yolk sac (Rombough, 1988), is expected to be the most proficient gas exchange surface for a larval fish. Despite this, the O_2 map showed that the JO_2 across the yolk sac is not significantly different from the thicker and less vascularized trunk region, a result which was also shown by intravascular PO_2 measurements made in larval rainbow trout (Rombough, 1992). Furthermore, multi-chamber respirometry on salmonids revealed that the yolk sac is a less effective gas exchanger than the rest of the body (Rombough and Ure, 1991; Wells and Pinder, 1996b). In contrast, recent studies using SMOT have shown that JO_2 is higher at the yolk sac than at the trunk for larval zebrafish. However, in Hughes et al. (2019) and Zimmer et al. (2020), the JO_2 measured at the yolk sac may have reflected contributions from two major O_2 sinks (heart and developing gills) and thus biasing the comparison. Instead, if one considers Fig. 3D from Zimmer et al. (2020) and compares the JO_2 taken at points 4 and 6 on the yolk sac and the trunk respectively, the JO_2 is not significantly different. The presence of a significant anterior-to-posterior trend of cutaneous JO_2 illustrated by

Figures 2B and 5B and recent work by Parker et al. (2020) highlights the importance of correcting for position when comparing JO_2 of two points on along the body surface.

The areas of highest JO_2 on the epithelium were found around the pectoral fins of the larva. It was found by Zimmer et al. (2020) that the pectoral fins aid in the dissipation of boundary layers on the surface of larval rainbow trout but the effect is not as clear with larval zebrafish. Considering that boundary layer PO_2 gradients have been considered the most significant resistance for cutaneous O_2 uptake (Rombough, 1988), it is surprising that given the close proximity of the larval zebrafish pectoral fins to the major O_2 sinks of the body, there was no impact of removing the pectoral fins on the PO_2 gradients of the skin (Zimmer et al. 2020).

2.5.2 Cutaneous JO_2 patterns through development

Although this study looked at only two developmental time points of the larval zebrafish (4 and 7 dpf), already, notable differences in cutaneous JO_2 were observed. At 4 dpf, combined JO_2 (Fig. 2.2C) appears significantly higher than at 7 dpf (Fig. 2.5C). Despite this, the magnitude of $\dot{M}O_2$ does not differ significantly between the two ages. It appears that posterior JO_2 remained unchanged as the larvae aged with the major decrease in JO_2 occurring in the anterior and a slight decrease within the middle region (Figs. 2.2B and 2.5B). As vascularity does not appear to significantly change between 4 dpf and 7 dpf (Fig. 2.8), the age-dependent changes in JO_2 may be due to a thickening of the epithelium which would slow down O_2 diffusion according to Fick's Law and thus decrease JO_2. Further work remains to be done to determine the water-to-blood diffusion distance.

2.5.3 Compensatory mechanisms during hypoxia-exposure and their impact on cutaneous JO_2

The physical properties of an aquatic environment cause a challenge to O_2 movement and therefore, the physiological adaptations of fish to hypoxia have been well-documented. For larval zebrafish, hypoxia exposure leads to an increased number of O_2-sensing neuroepithelial cells on the skin (Dean et al., 2017), increased vascularity and blood vessel diameter (Moore et al., 2006; Schwerte, 2003), and altered gene regulation of major metabolic pathways (Köblitz et al., 2015; Robertson et al., 2014). Moreover, a prior exposure of 4 dpf zebrafish to hypoxia or anoxia led larvae to sustain O_2 uptake at a lower PO_2 which is indicative of an increased hypoxia performance (Robertson et al., 2014). The results of Chapter 2 reveal that after a pre-exposure to hypoxia, the JO_2 profile of the epithelium was not markedly different (Figs 2.1, 2.2, 2.4 and 2.5). This result was not predicted given the documented, acclimatory adjustments that larval zebrafish exhibit under hypoxia. Despite this it may be that the results found within the literature can only be observed after an exposure to a lower PO_2 than that used in this study. At 4 dpf, there was no difference in $\dot{M}O_2$ between normoxia- and hypoxia-exposed WT, result which is also recorded by Robertson et al. (2014). In contrast, there was a difference at 7 dpf with hypoxic-treated larvae displaying a lower $\dot{M}O_2$. This differs from Mandic et al. (2020) which saw no difference. The differences between the studies could be explained by the different types of hypoxia exposures that were used. Robertson et al. (2014) used 8 mmHg as the hypoxia exposure, a more severe treatment than the 40 mmHg exposure used in this study. In addition, Mandic et al. (2020) used longer hypoxia exposures of 1 days and 3 days at 30 and 90 mmHg respectively. The discrepancy highlights the importance of considering hypoxia exposure parameters when comparing results from different studies.

Finally, to help explain any potential changes in cutaneous JO_2 or P_{crit} after hypoxia pre-exposure, trunk vascularity of 4 and 7 dpf larvae was determined (Fig. 2.8). A vascularization index was calculated by multiplying total vessel length and number of vessel junctions because an increase in these parameters would theoretically lead to an increased surface of exchange for O_2 diffusion and thus potentially lead to increased JO_2. In addition, an increase in the number of junctions suggests an increased complexity and connectivity to the vascular system. Initially, it was predicted that vascularity would increase after WTs were exposed to hypoxia as has been previously shown in 6 dpf larval zebrafish (Yaqoob and Schwerte, 2010). However, there was no difference in vascularity index at 4 or 7 dpf. This result supports data from the JO_2 maps (Figs. 2.1 and 2.4) as JO_2 was unaffected by prior exposure to hypoxia. Notably, at 4 dpf Yaqoob and Schwerte (2010) also did not find a difference in vascularity between normoxia- and hypoxia-exposed larvae. The discrepancy arises when comparing 7 dpf larvae, at which time a significant difference was found by Yaqoob and Schwerte (2010). This difference may be explained by the more severe and longer duration hypoxia exposure of 20 mmHg for 48h used by Yaqoob and Schwerte (2010). Additionally, different techniques for measuring vascularity were used in two studies and have yet to be compared.

2.5.4 The role of Hif-1α in mediating regional O_2 uptake after hypoxia exposure

Hif-1α is the major regulator of cellular processes under hypoxia (Benita et al., 2009; Iyer et al., 1998) and has been linked to increased hypoxia tolerance o in zebrafish larvae pre-exposed to hypoxia (Mandic et al., 2020). Despite this evidence, the O_2 map of Hif-1α double-knockout larvae was not significantly different from the other treatments, especially that of WT larvae which were pre-exposed to hypoxia (Figs 2.2A and 2.5A). It was expected that the WT larvae pre-exposed to hypoxia would display a greater capacity for O_2 uptake due to the Hif-1α cascade of hypoxia-induced responses (including angiogenesis) while the knockout line would not be able to benefit and therefore JO_2 across the epithelium of the mutants would be unchanged.

Using micro-respirometry, whole-body $\dot{M}O_2$ was determined. There was an effect of genotype at 4 dpf with WT larvae displaying a greater $\dot{M}O_2$ than Hif1aa$^{-/-}$ab$^{-/-}$ larvae (Fig. 2.3A). This effect may be due to an early developmental delay caused by the knockout of Hif-1α as by 7 dpf WT (normoxia) and Hif1aa$^{-/-}$ab$^{-/-}$ (normoxia) show no difference in $\dot{M}O_2$ (Fig. 2.6A). In addition, hypoxia-treated larvae at 7 dpf exhibited a significantly decreased $\dot{M}O_2$.

To determine hypoxia tolerance, P_{crit} was measured. It was predicted that P_{crit} in the mutant larvae would show an unchanged P_{crit} between normoxia- and hypoxia-exposed, an effect which was observed both at 4 and 7 dpf (Figs. 2.3B and 2.6B). Consequently, Hif1aa$^{-/-}$ab$^{-/-}$ P_{crit} was also not different from that of WT 4 dpf larvae which suggests Hif-1α knockout does not affect hypoxia performance at this age. In contrast, Hif1aa$^{-/-}$ab$^{-/-}$ P_{crit} was different from that of 7 dpf WT which provides evidence to support the role of Hif-1α in mediating hypoxia performance.

Finally, as Hif-1α was shown to play a key role in angiogenesis (Gerri et al., 2017) it was predicted that WTs would exhibit increased vascularity which would be reduced in knockout larvae. Indeed, there was no difference in the vascularity index of Hif1aa$^{-/-}$ab$^{-/-}$ larvae at both 4 dpf and 7 dpf (Fig. 2.8). Despite this, the vascularity of WT larvae did not differ from that of Hif1aa$^{-/-}$ab$^{-/-}$ larvae and thus, this suggests that Hif-1α plays a minor role in regulating angiogenesis of the trunk vasculature at 4 and 7 dpf under the given hypoxia treatment.

2.5.5 Summary

The results of this study show that cutaneous JO_2 can vary substantially across the cutaneous surface of 4 and 7 dpf larval zebrafish. There is a strong regional effect of cutaneous JO_2 with the greatest flux taking place around the head and pectoral fin of the larva. One of the two major goals of the study was to evaluate the impact of previous hypoxia exposure on cutaneous O_2 uptake. It was shown that hypoxia exposure at 40 mmHg had no effect on cutaneous JO_2 in larvae at 4 and 7 dpf, a finding which is supported by data on trunk vascularity which also remained unchanged. Ultimately, the fall in P_{crit} in 7 dpf hypoxia pre-exposed larvae cannot be explained by an increase in vascularity. The second major goal of the study was to evaluate the role of Hif-1α in mediating cutaneous O_2 uptake. Similarly, the results of this study suggest that epithelial O_2 transfer is unaffected by the knockout of Hif-1α even after exposure to hypoxia. This study provides meaningful insight into O_2 uptake of a larval fish through the combination of regional JO_2 measurements facilitated by SMOT and $\dot{M}O_2$ through micro-respirometry which was used to address important questions of respiratory physiology such as the effect of hypoxia exposure and the role of Hif-1α.

Chapter 3

Parker, J. J., Zimmer, A. M. and Perry, S. F. (2020). Respirometry and cutaneous oxygen flux measurements reveal a negligible aerobic cost of ion regulation in larval zebrafish (*Danio rerio*). *J. Exp. Biol.*

Conceptualization: A.M.Z., S.F.P.; Methodology: J.J.P., A.M.Z.; Validation: J.J.P., A.M.Z.; Formal analysis: J.J.P.; Investigation: J.J.P.; Resources: S.F.P.; Data curation: J.J.P.; Writing - original draft: J.J.P.; Writing - review & editing: A.M.Z., S.F.P.; Supervision: A.M.Z., S.F.P.; Project administration: S.F.P.; Funding acquisition: S.F.P.

3.1 INTRODUCTION

For most fishes, maintaining and regulating internal ion balance is essential for survival. Many adaptations exist in freshwater (FW) and seawater (SW) fishes to counteract the ionic challenges of their native environments. Most FW teleost fishes are hyperionic and hyperosmotic relative to their external environment. These ionic and osmotic differences favour the passive loss of ions by diffusion and the continual gain of water through osmosis (Evans et al., 2005). To combat ion loss, FW teleost fishes absorb Na^+, Cl^- and Ca^{2+} across cutaneous (larvae) and branchial (adults) epithelia using specialized, mitochondrion-rich cells termed ionocytes. Depending on subtype (see below), ionocytes express specific channels, exchangers and ATP-dependent transporters to facilitate ion uptake (Dymowska et al., 2012; Evans, 2011; Evans and Claiborne JB, 2009; Evans et al., 2005; Gilmour and Perry, 2009; Guh et al., 2015; Hwang, 2009; Hwang, 2010; Hwang and Chou, 2013; Hwang and Lee, 2007; Hwang and Lin, 2013; Hwang and Perry, 2010; Hwang et al., 2011; Marshall, 2002; Marshall et al., 2006; Perry and Gilmour, 2006; Perry et al., 2003). The metabolic demands of these cells are presumed to be high owing to the abundance of mitochondria and ATP-consuming transporters (Dymowska et al., 2012; Zikos et al., 2014). However, currently there is no consensus on the metabolic costs of ion regulation in FW fishes.

Indeed, comprehensive reviews of the literature (Bœuf and Payan, 2001; Ern et al., 2014; Kirschner, 1995) suggest cost estimates ranging from less than a percent to 50% of metabolic rate (MR) for FW fishes. A common method for determining estimates has been to compare salinity-related differences in metabolism for a given species with the assumption that osmoregulatory costs are close to zero within an iso-osmotic environment. Using this method, costs for rainbow trout (*Oncorhynchus mykiss*) in FW was 20% of MR (Rao, 1968), 19% for the

Nile tilapia (*Oreochromis niloticus*; Farmer and Beamish, 1969), 50% for the brown bullhead (*Ameiurus nebulosus*; Furspan et al., 1984), "negligible" for the striped mullet (*Mugil cephalus*; Nordlie and Leffler, 1975) and potentially less than 12.5% of MR for the European perch (*Perca fluviatilis*; Christensen et al., 2017).

In contrast, studies which used theoretical models for determining osmoregulatory costs have estimated much lower costs. For example, by measuring the rate of total ion uptake, the electrical gradient between the water and blood of the fish and the resting metabolic rate (RMR), Eddy (1982) estimated that 1% of RMR of FW rainbow trout (*Oncorhynchus mykiss*) and less than 4 % of BMR in goldfish (*Carassius auratus*) was attributed to osmoregulation. Moreover, these results are supported by another model presented by Kirschner (1995) which concluded that rainbow trout allocate less than 2% of MR for osmoregulation in FW. Finally, a study that examined the O_2 consumption of excised gills from FW-adapted cutthroat trout (*Oncorhynchus clarkii*) found that following exposure to bafilomycin A1 and ouabain (H^+ ATPase and Na^+/K^+ ATPase inhibitors, respectively), gill tissue O_2 consumption dropped by 37%. This was translated to a 1.8% cost of whole animal O_2 uptake dedicated to NaCl uptake (Morgan and Iwama, 1999).

Not only is there a wide range in the current estimates of the metabolic cost of ionic regulation in fishes, to our knowledge, there are no data concerning such costs in larval stages. The ionoregulatory mechanisms underlying the absorption of Na^+, Cl^- and Ca^{2+} uptake in zebrafish larvae have been extensively investigated and are summarised in a number of comprehensive reviews (Evans, 2011; Guh et al., 2015; Hwang, 2009; Hwang and Lee, 2007; Hwang and Perry, 2010; Hwang et al., 2011; Kumai and Perry, 2012). In particular, the Na^+ uptake pathways in larval zebrafish are well characterised and share the reliance on basolateral

Na^+/K^+ ATPase for ultimate entry into the blood. Basolateral Na^+/K^+ ATPase activity is considered a central contributor to the ionoregulatory costs in FW fishes (Kirschner, 1995). Three apical pathways for Na^+ transport in zebrafish larvae are proposed; i) electroneutral Na^+/H^+ exchange via a Na^+/H^+-exchanger 3b (Nhe3b; *slc9a3.2*) (Esaki et al., 2007) ii) H^+-ATPase (HA) activity linked with a putative epithelial Na^+ channel (potentially an acid-sensing ion channel) (Dymowska et al., 2015; Zimmer et al., 2018) and iii) Na^+-Cl^- cotransport (NCC) facilitated by *slc12a10.2* (Wang et al., 2009). The NHE3b- and HA-facilitated pathways are expressed in HA-rich cells (HRC) and the NCC mediated pathway resides in NCC ionocytes (Guh et al., 2015). The contribution of each pathway may differ depending on the prevailing environmental conditions (Hwang and Lee, 2007a; Shih et al., 2012; Yan et al., 2007). Notably, Na^+ uptake capacity in zebrafish larvae is increased markedly upon or after exposure to waters of low pH or low Na^+ content (Kumai and Perry, 2011; Kumai et al., 2011; Kwong and Perry, 2016; Shih et al., 2012). Such increases in Na^+ uptake are expected to increase metabolic cost given the active nature of Na^+ uptake.

The aim of this study was to determine the aerobic costs associated with Na^+ regulation in larval zebrafish. It was hypothesized that changes in the rate of Na^+ uptake would significantly influence the O_2 consumption of the Na^+-transporting ionocytes and thus affect whole body $\dot{M}O_2$ as well as cutaneous O_2 flux at the yolk sac owing to its high density of ionocytes. In addition to exploiting the naturally occurring spatial distribution of cutaneous ionocytes, this hypothesis was tested using an integrated approach whereby rates of Na^+ uptake were manipulated and/or ionocyte numbers altered by exposing fish to low Na^+ or acidic water and after morpholino knockdown of Foxi3a [transcription factor responsible for ionocyte specification and differentiation (Hsiao et al., 2007)] or optical ablation of HR cells.

3.2 MATERIAL AND METHODS

3.2.1 Zebrafish

Wild-type (WT) zebrafish (*Danio rerio*) were housed at the University of Ottawa aquatic care facility. Fish were maintained in plastic aquaria which were constantly supplied with aerated, dechloraminated City of Ottawa tap water at 28°C (referred to as "system water"; in mM: 0.25 Ca^{2+}, 0.78 Na^{+}, 0.4 Cl^{-}, 0.025 K^{+}, 0.15 Mg^{2+}; pH 7.6). Fish were kept on a 14 h light: 10 h dark photoperiod and fed until satiation with no. 1 crumble-Zeigler (Aquatic Habitats; Apoka, FL) once a day. Unless otherwise stated, for all experiments, zebrafish at 4 days post fertilisation (dpf) were used. Larvae were obtained by breeding adult zebrafish in plastic 2 L breeding traps with a perforated insert. For breeding, 8 – 10 fish at a ratio of 2 females to 1 male were placed in breeding traps and left overnight. The following morning, embryos were collected using a fine mesh sieve and were placed in 50 mL petri dishes at a density of 30 embryos per dish containing different media, based on experimental protocols (see below), and held in an incubator set to 28.5°C. Media in the petri dishes was replaced daily until experimentation at 4 dpf. All experiments were conducted in compliance with the Canadian Council of Animal Care guidelines and after approval of the University of Ottawa Animal Care Committee (protocols BL-2118 and BL-1700).

3.2.2 Scanning micro-optrode technique (SMOT)

Experiments were designed to detect local JO_2 at the yolk sac epithelium of 4 dpf larval zebrafish in response to various experimental manipulations (see Experimental Series below) using SMOT (Hughes et al., 2019; Zimmer et al., 2020). The purpose of the JO_2 measures was to provide a direct assessment of the aerobic metabolism of the ionocytes with the highest resolution possible with current available techniques. The SMOT system consists of a fibre optic oxygen optrode (PreSens Precision Sensing GmbH, Regensburg, Germany) connected to a detector system and motion control unit developed by Applicable Electronics (Science Wares, Inc., Falmouth, MA, USA). Oxygen optrodes were constructed from fiber optic cables that were flame-pulled to a 40 μm tip and coated with Pt(II) meso-Tetra(pentafluorophenyl)porphyrin (Pt-TFPP; Frontier Scientific, Newark, DE, USA). The optrode was connected to the detector system that emits an excitation light through a blue LED ($\lambda = 400$ nm) that excites the Pt-TFPP coating and detects fluorescence emission. The fluorescent emission from Pt-TFPP is quenched in the presence of oxygen. The position of the optrode was manipulated using an Applicable Electronics CMC-4 (Applicable Electronics, New Haven, CT, USA) computer motion control unit and recordings were measured using ASET-LV4 software (Applicable Electronics).

To apply SMOT, a setup in which fish could be secured in place was necessary. Larvae (2 - 4 dpf, depending on the experimental series) were anaesthetised, individually, in a solution of 0.20 mg mL^{-1} tricaine methane sulfonate (MS-222; Syndel Laboratories Ltd., Nanaimo, BC, Canada) buffered to pH 7.6 for 5 min. Tricaine used in low doses as in this study does not affect O_2 consumption in chinook salmon (*Oncorhynchus tshawytscha*) larvae but does prevent pectoral and opercular movements (Rombough, 1988). Afterwards, fish were transferred to a modified Petri dish (Hughes et al., 2019) filled with the appropriate treatment solution, depending on the experimental series. The modified dish contained a thin bottom layer of Sylgard 184 silicon elastomer (Dow Corning, Midland, MI, USA). A thin strap of Sylgard was placed over the tail of the larva, with both ends of the strap secured to the bottom of the dish with Austerlitz 0.20 mm minutiens insect pins (Entomoravia, Slakov u Brna, Czech Republic). The head of the larva was secured in place against a second, thicker strip of Sylgard that acted as a buttress (Hughes et al.,

2019). This method of securing the larva in place was necessary because initial experiments demonstrated that the larva would otherwise drift as the probe moved during measurements. To ensure that measurements were made at ionocyte-expressing epithelia, larvae were vitally stained with 1 μM MitoTracker CMXRos Red (MitoROS; ThermoFisher, Burlington, ON, Canada) for 10 min and 0.05 mg mL^{-1} of Concanavalin A (ConA), a lectin that binds specifically to HR cells of zebrafish larvae (Lin et al., 2006), conjugated to Alexa 488 (ThermoFisher) for 30 min. A control experiment designed to test the effect of the cell stains on cutaneous JO_2 was performed by measuring JO_2 across the yolk sac extension of stained and unstained larvae. No statistically significant effect was found ($n = 5$; $p = 0.154$, Fig. S1).

Before each experiment, the optrode was calibrated in zero solution (20 g/L anhydrous Na_2SO_3) and air-saturated media that matched the corresponding experimental series. SMOT measurements were conducted by initially positioning the optrode directly above (5 -10 μm) the epithelium of the yolk sac. The first measurement of O_2 partial pressure (PO_2) was taken at this location. The probe was then set to follow an excursion distance of 100 μm in the z-plane to take the second measurement. Measurements were recorded for 2 sec followed by a waiting period of 5 sec. This was repeated five times for each specific point on the epithelium; time between replicates was set to 10 sec. For all experiments, PO_2 was measured at three equidistant points along the yolk sac extension (area where ionocytes are present) and at three adjacent points along the posterior trunk (area where ionocytes are absent) for a single larva ($n = 1$). Observations were made using a Nikon SMZ 1500 (Nikon Instruments, Melville, NY, U.S.A.) fluorescence dissection microscope.

Fick's law of diffusion was used to calculate oxygen flux (JO_2; pmol cm^{-2} s^{-1}) based on the following equation:

$$JO_2 = -D((dPO_2 * \alpha O_2)/dx) \qquad (1)$$

where D is the oxygen diffusion coefficient ($2.2 * 10^{-5}$ cm s^{-1}) in water at 25°C (Ferrell et al. 1967), dPO_2 (mm Hg) is the difference in PO_2 measured along the 100 μm excursion distance, αO_2 is the O_2 solubility constant (1.5906 pmol cm^{-3} $mmHg^{-1}$) in water at 25°C (Boutilier et al. 1984), and dx (cm) is the excursion distance of the probe. For each fish, a five replicate, background dPO_2 was measured approximately 3 cm away from the larva and was subtracted from the experimental dPO_2.

3.2.3 Microrespirometry

Whole-body O_2 consumption was measured in 2 or 4 dpf larvae to complement the localized measurements of JO_2 using SMOT. The system (Loligo Systems, Viborg, Denmark) consisted of a 24-well, glass microplate in which each chamber had a volume of 80 μL (well inner diameter d = 4.5 mm). Each well contained a non-invasive O_2 sensor spot, which was scanned by a 24-channel optical fluorescence O_2 microplate reader. The microplate was placed in a temperature-controlled (29.9 °C) water bath held on a shaker (continuous circular oscillations set to 30 RPM with a deviation of 25 mm) to prevent the formation of unstirred layers of water surrounding each larva. The sensors were calibrated using zero solution and air-saturated water (see above) after sealing the microplate using PCR tape, a silicone pad and a compression block. Care was taken to remove air bubbles from the wells before recording PO_2. Following calibration, wells were rinsed thoroughly and larvae from each respective treatment were assigned randomly to wells (1 larva per well). PO_2 was recorded continuously for approximately 30 min.

O_2 consumption ($\dot{M}O_2$; pmol mg^{-1} h^{-1}) was calculated using the following equation:

$$\dot{M}O_2 = (dPO_2 * \alpha O_2 * V)/m \quad (2)$$

where dPO_2 is the rate of change of PO_2 (mm Hg h^{-1}) within the chamber over time, αO_2 is the O_2 solubility constant (pmol L^{-1} mm Hg^{-1}) in water at 30 °C (Boutilier et al., 1984), V is the volume (L) of the chamber and m is the average mass of the larva (mg). For the 2 dpf larvae (see below), rates were expressed on a per larva basis because they were too small to be weighed accurately. Wet mass was determined by placing 40 X 4 dpf larvae (anaesthetized by placing on ice) in a small, pre-weighed insert lined with a fine mesh, which was fixed atop a 50 mL falcon tube. To remove excess water, the bottom of the mesh was blotted with a tissue and then centrifuged at 400 rpm for 1 min. The fine mesh cup containing the larvae was then reweighed on an analytic balance to obtain the mass of the pool of 40 larvae (n = 1), which was used to estimate individual mass of the larva in the respirometer.

3.2.4 Na^+ uptake

To calculate Na^+ uptake, 12 larvae were placed in 2 mL centrifuge tubes containing 1.6 mL of experimental media, depending on the experimental series (see below) in a 29 °C water bath (a previously performed experiment showed that oxygen levels in the 2 mL tube did not fall below 80% over a 3 h incubation period - data not shown). After larvae were allowed to settle for 30 min, $^{22}Na^+$ was added to each tube (0.4 μCi/tube for 4 dpf larvae assayed in normal Na^+ (N-Na), 0.05 μCi/tube for 4 dpf larvae assayed in low Na^+ (L-Na), 0.8 μCi/tube for 2 dpf larvae assayed in N-Na; see Experimental Series), marking the beginning of the flux period. Fish were incubated with $^{22}Na^+$ for 3 h, with 0.7 mL water samples collected at 0 and 3 h, after which fish were euthanized with neutralized MS-222 and rinsed 4 X in 10 mmol L^{-1} NaCl to displace any loosely bound $^{22}Na^+$. Larvae were collected in pairs (n =1) into centrifuge tubes. $^{22}Na^+$ gamma-radioactivity in paired larvae and water samples was measured by gamma-counting (2470

Wizard2, Perkin Elmer, Waltham, MA, USA) and Na^+ concentration of water samples was measured by atomic absorption flame spectrophotometry (Spectra AA 220FS, Varian, Palo Alto, CA). Na^+ uptake (pmol mg^{-1} h^{-1}) was calculated using the equation:

$$Na^+ \text{ uptake} = R_{larvae}/SA/t/n/m \quad (3)$$

where R_{larvae} is the gamma radioactivity (cpm) present in the paired larval sample, SA is the specific activity (cpm $pmol^{-1}$) of the water, t is flux duration (h), *n* is the number of larvae in the counted sample which was always two, and m was the individual weight (mg) for a larva from the respective treatment group. For the 2 dpf larvae, rates were expressed on a per larva basis because they were too small to be weighed accurately.

3.2.5 Ionocyte density

Larvae were observed under a Nikon SMZ 1500 microscope equipped with the 49008 - ET – mcherry, Texas Red® filter cube set (Chroma Technology Corp, Bellow Falls, VT, USA) and images of the fluorescently stained, apical surface of the yolk sac were captured using a 1.3-megapixel CMOS sensor connected to µEYE cockpit software (iDS; Obersulm, Germany). Cells were counted manually, and surface area of the yolk sac was determined by Image-J 1.51 open source software (National Institutes of Health, Bethesda, MD, USA). Epithelial JO_2 was measured across the yolk sac of each larvae. A correlation analysis was performed to determine relatedness by plotting MR cell density (x-axis) against JO_2 (y-axis).

In our initial studies, it was found that JO_2 was lowest near the yolk sac extension. Thus, all subsequent SMOT measurements were performed across the yolk sac extension because the lower "background" JO_2 would allow for greater sensitivity to detect changes in JO_2 resulting from metabolic changes in ionocytes.

2.3.6 Manipulation of water chemistry

Zebrafish were reared in reconstituted media resembling system water, composed of the following constituents (in mM): 0.15 $MgSO_4 \cdot 7H_2O$, 0.02 K_2HPO_4 , 0.05 KH_2PO_4, 0.25 $CaCl_2$, 0.4 Na_2SO_4; pH 7.6. Unless otherwise mentioned, larvae were reared under N-Na conditions (800 μM) and maintained at pH 7.6. Rearing media was titrated daily to pH 7.6 using dilute KOH or H_2SO_4 and was replaced daily. In one experiment, larvae were reared in N-Na adjusted to pH 4 (low pH; L-pH) using H_2SO_4 and were acutely transferred to pH 7.6 at 4 dpf, just prior to experimentation. In a second experiment, larvae reared in N-Na were acutely transferred to L-Na conditions (5 μM Na^+; 2.5 μM Na_2SO_4) just prior to experimentation and a separate group of larvae were reared in L-Na and acutely transferred to N-Na conditions prior to experimentation. Na^+ uptake, whole-body respirometry, and SMOT measurements were performed on larvae from all treatments.

3.2.7 Foxi3a morpholino knockdown

Knockdown of the transcription factor *foxi3a* (NCBI reference sequence: NM_198917.2) was used to prevent ionocyte differentiation in larvae (Hsiao et al., 2007). However, the effect of *foxi3a* knockdown lasted only until 2 dpf (unpublished observations) and therefore experiments on *foxi3a* morphants (individuals experiencing morpholino knockdown) were performed at 2 dpf. Knockdown was achieved by the microinjection of an antisense morpholino oligonucleotide. Embryos were injected at the 1-cell stage with 4 ng of either a sham morpholino (5'-CCTCTTACCTCAGTTACAATTTATA-3'; Gene Tools, Philomath, OR, USA) that has no biological target in zebrafish or a morpholino targeting the translation start site of *foxi3a* (5'-CCTTCAACAAAGAGAAACGGGGAAGA-3' (Hsiao et al., 2007); Gene Tools) suspended in 1 nL of Danieau buffer (in mM: 58 NaCl, 0.7 KCl, 0.4 $MgSO_4$, 0.6 $Ca(NO_3)_2$, and 5.0 Hepes; pH

7.6) containing 0.05% phenol red for visualization. At 2 dpf, zebrafish were dechorionated with fine forceps prior to Na^+ uptake, microrespirometry, and SMOT measurements. After 2 dpf, ionocyte density in *foxi3a* morphants gradually increased across the larval yolk sac. The sparsely spaced ionocytes accommodated the tip of the SMOT probe and made it possible to make flux measurements over areas where ionocytes were present or absent on the yolk sac extension.

3.2.8 Cell ablation

Larvae at 4 dpf reared under N-Na and pH 7.6 were stained with MitoRos and ConA and then anaesthetised in a solution of 0.20 mg mL^{-1} MS-222. Larvae were embedded at room temperature with 1.8% low-melting point agar (Bioshop Canada Inc., Burlington, ON, Canada) in the bottom of a 10 mm Petri dish. After the agar solidified, the Petri dish was filled with MS-222-containing N-Na water and the larvae were examined using a single-photon, scanning confocal laser microscope ($A1R^+$, Nikon Instruments, Melville, NY, USA). A 404.6 nm laser set to 100 % power was used to ablate patches of ionocytes along the yolk sac extension; ablation was confirmed visually by the absence of fluorescence in the ablated areas. Exposure time was set to 32.2 sec and scan speed was set to 1/32. These settings were shown previously to successfully ablate melanocytes on larval zebrafish (Yang et al., 2004) . Following cell ablation, larvae were removed from the agar bed using fine forceps and left to recover for 30 min in fresh reconstituted water prior to SMOT measurements.

3.2.9 Statistical analyses

All statistical analyses were performed using SigmaPlot (version 11.0; Systat Software, Chicago, IL, USA). Data are reported as means ± standard error of the mean (s.e.m.). Statistical significance of treatment effects was evaluated through two-way and one-way analysis of variance (ANOVA) followed by a Holm-Sidak *post-hoc* test or a Student's t-test. Statistical significance was accepted at $P \leq 0.05$. Specific details of statistical analyses are included in corresponding figure captions.

3.3 RESULTS

3.3.1 JO_2 at the yolk sac and trunk of 4 dpf larval zebrafish

Epithelial JO_2 was measured within three regions of the yolk sac (Fig. 3.1A) near small clusters of MR cells (Fig. 3.1B). The regions were arbitrarily designated as follows: anterior (region anterior to the apex of the yolk sac), middle (posterior to the apex of the yolk sac, but anterior to the yolk sac extension), and posterior (yolk sac extension). MR density (including HR density) was determined for each larva. MR density was significantly lower in the posterior portion of the yolk sac but was not significantly different for HR cells across the yolk sac (Fig. 3.2A). Furthermore, the posterior region also displayed the lowest JO_2, revealing a declining anterior-to-posterior trend in JO_2 along the yolk sac (Fig. 3.2B), however, there was no relationship ($R^2 = 0.006$) between JO_2 and ionocyte density across the yolk sac (Fig. 3.2C).

3.3.2 Effects of L-pH and L-Na rearing conditions

Larvae were reared in normal (pH 7.6; mass = 0.2205 mg ± 0.0122 mg, n = 9) or low (pH 4; mass = 0.2489 mg ± 0.0253 mg, n = 6) pH conditions but were transferred to pH 7.6 immediately prior to Na^+ uptake, $\dot{M}O_2$ or JO_2 measurements. Na^+ uptake rate was significantly higher in larvae that were reared in pH 4, however, $\dot{M}O_2$ was significantly lower (Fig. 3.3A, B). JO_2 at the yolk sac extension or trunk was not significantly affected by L-pH acclimation (Fig. 3.3C).

In response to acute transfer from N-Na to L-Na conditions, Na^+ uptake rate was significantly reduced, but was stimulated in larvae reared in L-Na conditions (mass = 0.2409 mg ± 0.246 mg, n = 6) and transferred to N-Na conditions (Fig. 3.4A). Despite these changes in Na^+ uptake rates, $\dot{M}O_2$ (Fig. 3.4B) and JO_2 (Fig. 3.4C) measured under the same conditions were not significantly different across treatment groups. JO_2 was not significantly different between the yolk sac extension and trunk under any of the conditions (Fig. 3.4C).

3.3.3 Effect of *foxi3a* knockdown

At 2 dpf, ionocytes were present across the yolk sac extension of the sham larvae (Fig. 3.5A), but not the *foxi3a* morphants (Fig. 3.5B). This led to a large reduction in Na^+ uptake compared to the sham larvae (Fig. 3.6A). However, whole-body $\dot{M}O_2$ (Fig. 3.6B) and JO_2 (Fig. 3.6C) were not affected by *foxi3a* knockdown. Interestingly, a significant difference between JO_2 measured at the yolk sac extension and trunk was detected in 2 dpf larvae, but this difference was unaffected by *foxi3a* knockdown (Fig. 3.6C).

Noticeably, at 59 hours post-fertilization (hpf) ionocyte density on the yolk sac epithelium continued to increase for the sham larvae (Fig. 3.7A) and the morphants (Fig. 3.7B). At this age, regional JO_2 at sites with and without ionocytes was not significantly different (Fig. 3.7C).

3.3.4 Effect of ablating ionocytes on regional JO_2

Using single-photon confocal microscopy, cell ablation was carried out on the epithelium of 4 dpf larval zebrafish. Using Mitotracker staining as a guide (Fig. 3.8A), sites along the yolk sac extension were ablated (Fig. 3.8B) with the goal of destroying ionocytes while other sites were left unaffected. There were no significant differences in JO_2 between ablated and unablated sites across the yolk sac extension (Fig. 3.8C).

3.4 DISCUSSION

The purpose of this study was to assess the aerobic costs of Na^+ uptake in larval zebrafish. A major component of the experimental design consisted of manipulating water chemistry to increase or decrease the rate of Na^+ uptake. This protocol provided an opportunity to examine the relationship between Na^+ uptake rate and $\dot{M}O_2$/cutaneous JO_2 as well as cutaneous JO_2 at regions of low and high ionocyte abundance. Furthermore, through *foxi3a* knockdown, ionocyte differentiation was delayed causing a near elimination of Na^+ uptake. The results clearly demonstrated that $\dot{M}O_2$ and JO_2 were not correlated with rates of Na^+ uptake or ionocyte density, thereby demonstrating that Na^+ uptake does not incur measurable aerobic cost in zebrafish larvae. Ultimately, the findings of this study support the notion that ionic regulation incurs a relatively low aerobic cost in FW fishes (Eddy, 1982; Kirschner, 1995; Morgan and Iwama, 1999; Nordlie and Leffler, 1975).

It is important to acknowledge that the results of this study, strictly speaking, are valid only for zebrafish larvae (at 4 dpf) and may not necessarily apply to other species or other developmental stages, including adults. In rapidly developing larvae, growth presumably commands a significantly larger portion of the total energy budget in comparison to adults. Although it is conceivable that the high rates of anabolic processes in larvae masked the energetic costs of ionic regulation (Na^+ uptake), we consider this unlikely because the high rates of $\dot{M}O_2$ in larvae are roughly matched by equally high rates of Na^+ uptake (compare Fig 3.3A from this study with Fig 7B in Zimmer and Perry, 2020). Thus, the ratio of Na^+ uptake to $\dot{M}O_2$ is more-or-less constant (3.4-4.4%) in larvae and adults (derived using $\dot{M}O_2$ data from Fig 3.3B this study and Table 1 in Mandic et al., 2020). An additional caveat is that measuring $\dot{M}O_2$ using whole body respirometry may not necessarily reveal the true aerobic cost of ionic regulation if changes in O_2 consumption by ionocytes occurring during periods of experimentally altered Na^+ uptake are masked by reallocation of the energy budget such that overall $\dot{M}O_2$ remains unchanged. For this reason, the conclusions of the present study were heavily reliant on the results of the SMOT experiments in which measurements of JO_2 were localized to small clusters of ionocytes at the surface of the yolk sac epithelium and thus unaffected by the constraints of energy reallocation.

3.4.1 Ionocyte density does not significantly affect epithelial JO_2

Despite the finding of a decreasing ionocyte density (Fig. 3.2A) and a reduction in JO_2 (Fig. 3.2B) across the yolk sac in the anterior-to-posterior direction, the two factors were not correlated (Fig. 3.2C). Although boundary layer PO_2 can be an indicator for the regional O_2 demand of organisms such as rainbow trout larvae (Ciuhandu et al., 2007), our results demonstrate that epithelial JO_2 measured at the yolk sac surface was not influenced by ionocyte density. It is possible that the anterior-to-posterior trend in declining JO_2 was related to metabolic demand of underlying tissues or organs. For example, Hughes et al. (2019) reported that epithelial JO_2 in zebrafish larvae was highest around the heart/gill area and decreased towards the trunk. Thus, the higher JO_2 observed in the anterior yolk sac in the present study may have resulted from the underlying energetically demanding tissues, including the heart and developing gills. Additionally, given the reliance of JO_2 on blood flow (Hughes et al., 2019), the increased rates of JO_2 in the anterior region may reflect differences in perfusion.

3.4.2 Epithelial JO_2 is unaffected by altered Na^+ uptake capacity

Initial experiments (Fig. 3.2) suggested that ionocyte O_2 consumption was negligible under N-Na and pH 7.6. However, we predicted that under conditions that challenge Na^+ homeostasis, including exposure to L-pH or L-Na water, the aerobic demand of ionocytes might increase and thus be quantifiable using SMOT. Several changes to the ionoregulatory system occur under L-pH which would be expected to increase the metabolic demand of Na^+-transporting ionocytes. For example, HR cell density was shown to increase in 4 dpf zebrafish larvae acclimated to pH 4 water (Horng et al., 2009) and it follows that the increased number of mitochondrion-rich cells would lead to an increased O_2 demand. In addition, under chronic L-pH, HA mRNA and protein expression are increased (Chang et al., 2009; Horng et al., 2009; Lin et al., 2015; Yan et al., 2007), thus creating an increased demand for ATP to fuel the ATP-dependent transporter. Furthermore, L-pH rearing in zebrafish is accompanied by an increase in Na^+ uptake capacity (Kumai et al., 2011) that may be related to endocrine responses, leading to increased plasma levels of prolactin and cortisol that promote Na^+ uptake and increase HA activity (Kwong et al., 2014); these changes are assumed to come at an energetic cost to the larvae.

Thus, it was predicted that during periods of increased Na^+ uptake rate after exposure to L-pH, O_2 consumption and epithelial O_2 flux would increase. Despite stimulating Na^+ uptake capacity through the manipulation of environmental conditions, the results of microrespirometry and SMOT measurements did not support our hypothesis. Notably, under the L-pH treatment, $\dot{M}O_2$ was reduced (Fig. 3.3B) and epithelial JO_2 was unaffected (Fig. 3.3C) in larvae that had been reared in pH 4 and acutely transferred to pH 7.6, even though Na^+ uptake was significantly higher under these same conditions (Fig. 3.3A).

The discrepancy observed between whole-body $\dot{M}O_2$ and regional JO_2 may be linked to a slightly hindered development. Although considered an acid-tolerant species (Kwong et al., 2014), capable of surviving in pH 4.0 water, the ideal rearing pH for zebrafish is 6.8 – 7.5 (Avdesh et al., 2012). In light of the negative effects of acidic water exposure on the physiology of fishes (McDonald, 1983; Wood, 1989), it is possible that the L-pH environment negatively affected growth. Within the literature, it has been reported that zebrafish reared at pH 4.0 are marginally shorter (e.g. 6% shorter in the study of JavadiEsfahani and Kwong, 2019) or largely unaffected (Horng et al., 2007). Moreover, in this study larvae that were raised under pH 4.0 are slightly heavier than those raised under pH 7.6. Ultimately, the variation in body measures of pH 4.0 reared larvae prevents a conclusion which claims one specific causal factor. It must also be considered that although a change in growth or an impedance to the functioning of specific organs may alter O_2 consumption measured using whole-body microrespirometry it would not impact regional JO_2 measurements through SMOT as they are associated with small clusters of ionocytes.

Adult zebrafish acclimated to L-Na (0.04 mmol L^{-1} - Na^+) exhibited an increase in gill Na^+/H^+ exchanger 3b (NHE3b: *slc9a3b*) mRNA expression and a decrease in HA (*atp6v1aa*) mRNA expression (Yan et al., 2007). These results suggest that under L-Na, Na^+ uptake is managed principally by NHE3b in HR cells. Furthermore, using the scanning ion-selective electrode technique on 4 dpf zebrafish larvae, it was found that L-Na acclimation led to increased Na^+ uptake presumably by HR cells (Shih et al., 2012). These results suggest that the increase in Na^+ uptake observed in the current study in the L-Na acclimated larvae after acute transfer to N-Na, was a result of increased NHE3b activity. The acute reduction of ambient Na^+ accompanying the transfer of N-Na acclimated larvae to a L-Na environment caused a decrease in Na^+ uptake owing to less substrate being available to the Na^+/H^+ exchanger (Fig. 3.4A). Overall, despite these bidirectional alterations to Na^+ uptake, there were no accompanying differences in $\dot{M}O_2$ (Fig. 3.4B) or JO_2 (Fig. 3.4C) among the treatments. Thus, any changes in O_2 uptake of the ionocytes are negligible compared to the bulk O_2 uptake of the rest of the body.. Moreover, the fact that across all water chemistry conditions, there were no differences in JO_2 between the trunk (no ionocytes) and the yolk sac extension (abundant ionocytes) argues for an insignificant contribution of ionocytes to bulk O_2 flux (Figs. 3.3C and 3.4C). Again, however, it must be considered that the growth-dominant metabolism of the larvae may lead to an energetic reallocation when a reduction in ionoregulatory demands occurs

3.4.3 Manipulating ionocyte density did not affect $\dot{M}O_2$ or JO_2

To lower the energy expended on Na^+ uptake, ionocyte density was reduced experimentally (using *foxi3a* knockdown) to only a few scattered ionocytes across the whole-body (Fig. 3.5B). Owing to the elimination of O_2 uptake by the presumed metabolically active Na^+-transporting cells, it was predicted that the *foxi3a* knockdown would reveal reductions in whole-body and cutaneous O_2 uptake rates and that the reductions in cutaneous JO_2 would be restricted to the yolk sac. Despite the predicted fall in Na^+ uptake rate in the morphants compared to sham larvae (Fig. 3.6A), there was no difference in $\dot{M}O_2$ (Fig. 3.6B) or JO_2 (Fig. 3.6C), providing further evidence that the amount of energy utilized by the ionocytes is negligible. Notably, there was a significantly higher JO_2 at the trunk versus the yolk sac of two dpf larvae in both treatments (Fig. 3.6C), which may reflect a higher rate of O_2 consumption in the rapidly developing trunk relative to the yolk sac. However, this difference was not observed at other developmental stages nor was it observed in two previous studies that measured JO_2 in larvae at 4 dpf (Hughes et al., 2019; Zimmer et al., 2020). It is possible that differences in JO_2

between the trunk and yolk sac are greatest in the younger larvae (i.e. 2 dpf) when growth is presumably faster.

Subsequently, as ionocytes gradually developed at around 3 dpf, there was still no significant difference in JO_2 when measuring over sites with and without ionocytes (Fig. 3.7C). Considering that the larval epithelium consists of keratinocytes, mucous cells, club cells, ionocytes and undifferentiated cells (Chang and Hwang, 2011), it was reasonable to predict that sites with more mitochondrion-rich ionocytes would yield a higher JO_2 because the remaining mitochondrion-poor cell-types are assumed to have a lower energy requirement.

In addition to morpholino knockdown, cell ablation was used to reduce ionocyte density. Notably, it is likely that because ablation was non-specific, surrounding surface epithelial layers and deeper cell layers were also removed by the ablation. Despite this loss of cells, JO_2 was unaffected (Fig. 3.8C).

3.4.4 Perspectives and significance

In this study, the combinatorial approach of radioactive Na^+ tracing, whole-body microrespirometry and SMOT were used to assess the aerobic costs of Na^+ uptake in zebrafish larvae. Together, these techniques were complementary and allowed a thorough testing of the hypothesis. Through Na^+ tracing, it could be ensured that the larvae exhibited the predicted response in Na^+ uptake with specific treatments. Thus, the results from SMOT and whole-body microrespirometry could be interpreted with greater confidence. Notably, SMOT is a recently developed and technologically advanced technique (Ferreira et al., 2020) in this area of research and thus it was important to also implement a more tested technique such as whole body microrespirometry. Despite using arguably, the most sensitive technique available for measuring epithelial JO_2 in larval fishes, in addition to whole-body respirometry, the results of this study do not support the hypothesis that a substantial portion of aerobic metabolism is dedicated to ion regulation. It must be noted that this study was performed on larvae, which may have different metabolic demands compared to adults. However, even after a drastic reduction in ionocyte density leading to a near elimination of Na^+ uptake, there was no change in metabolic rate or oxygen flux. To date, the many studies that have assessed the metabolic costs associated with ionoregulation and osmoregulation in fishes have provided drastically different results, ranging from a negligible cost, to nearly 50% of metabolic rate. Our study supports the notion that the aerobic cost of Na^+ uptake and maintenance of ionocytes, at least in larvae, is negligible.

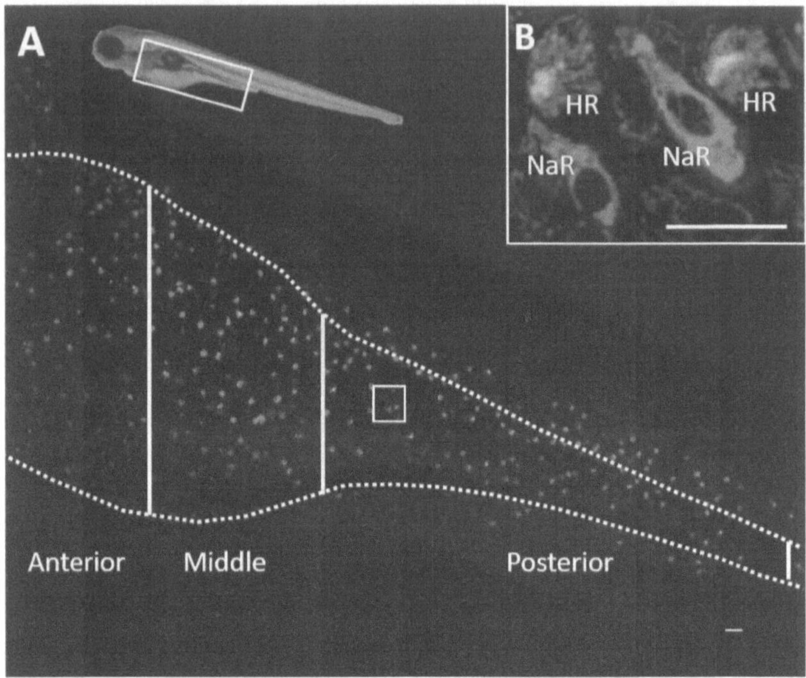

Figure. 3.1. Representative images of a MitoRos-stained (showing all MR cells) and ConA-stained (showing HR cells) 4 dpf larva (A-B). The arbitrary separation of anterior, middle and posterior sections of the yolk sac (contained within the dotted line) are shown (A) with a white square (not the exact same area as denoted in panel A but an enlarged image from a photo taken with an objective of higher magnification) within the posterior section highlighting a potential scan area for SMOT at a cluster of MR cells (B). Scale bars represent 20 microns.

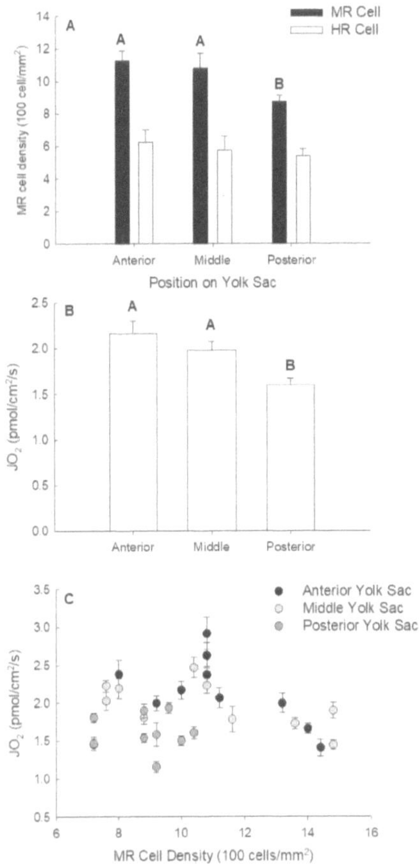

Figure 3.2. (A) Ionocyte density, (B) epithelial O_2 flux (JO_2) at the yolk sac, and (C) presentation of JO_2 as a function of ionocyte density in 4 dpf larval zebrafish. Larvae were reared and observed under N-Na and pH 7.6. Differing letters indicate statistically significant differences as determined by a one-way ANOVA followed by a Holm-Sidak post hoc analysis (A-B) (position: $p = 0.003$; $n = 9$). JO_2 at the yolk sac of 4 dpf zebrafish as a function of ionocyte density (C) ($R^2 = 0.006$; $n = 10$).

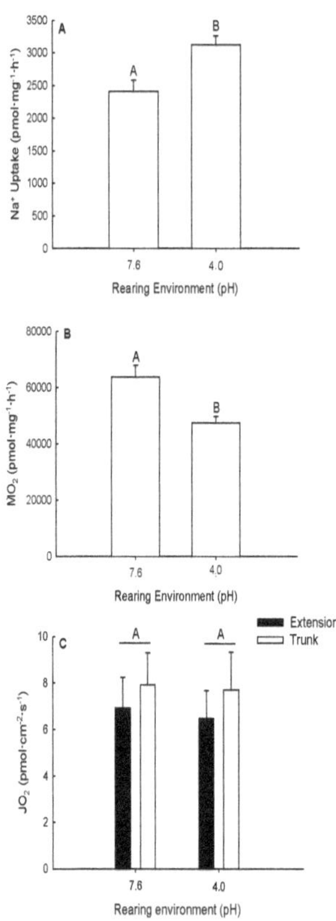

Figure. 3.3. The effects of L-pH on (A) Na^+ uptake, (B) whole-body O_2 consumption ($\dot{M}O_2$) and (C) epithelial O_2 flux (JO_2) in 4 dpf zebrafish. Larvae were reared in normal (pH 7.6) or acidic (pH 4) water but were all acutely transferred to pH 7.6 water prior to measurements. Differing letters denote a statistically significant effect of L-pH treatment as determined by a Student's t-test for Na^+ uptake ($p = 0.006$; $n = 8$) and $\dot{M}O_2$ ($p = 0.001$; $n = 19$-21). There were no significant effects of pH on JO_2 as determined by a two-way ANOVA followed by a Holm-Sidak post-hoc test (pH: $p = 0.797$; region: $p = 0.214$; interaction: $p = 0.571$; $n = 8$-9).

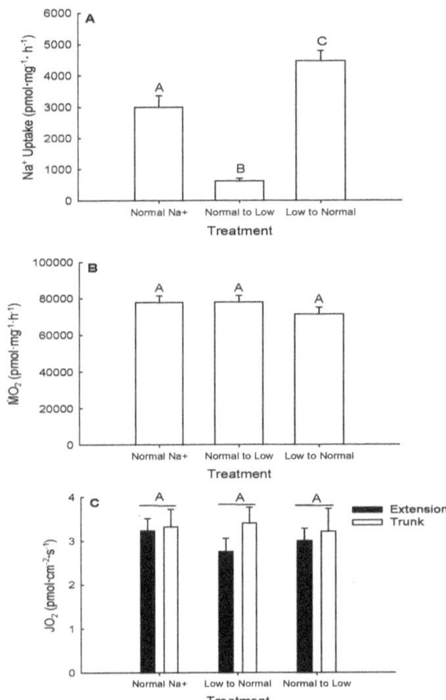

Figure 3.4. The effect of L-Na rearing and acute exposure on (A) Na^+ uptake, (B) whole-body $\dot{M}O_2$, and (C) epithelial JO_2 in 4 dpf zebrafish. Larvae were reared in N-Na water (800 μM) until 4 dpf and acutely transferred to either N-Na water ("Normal Na^+") or L-Na water (5 μM) ("Normal to Low") or were reared in L-Na water until 4 dpf and acutely transferred to N-Na water ("Low to Normal"). Differing letters indicate a significant difference between groups as analyzed using a one-way ANOVA followed by a Holm-Sidak post-hoc test for Na^+ uptake (treatment: $p < 0.05$; $n = 8$) and $\dot{M}O_2$ (treatment: $p = 0.344$. $n = 13$). There were no significant effects of Na^+ treatment on JO_2 as determined by a two-way ANOVA (Na^+: $p = 0.850$; region: $p = 0.305$; interaction: $p = 0.730$; $n = 5$).

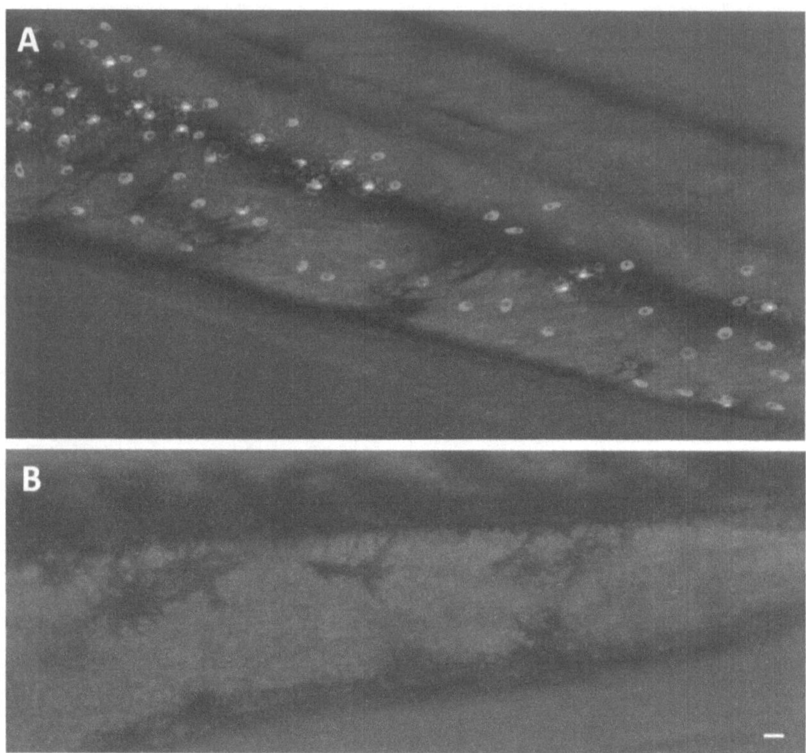

Figure 3.5. Representative images of (A) sham and (B) morphant 2 dpf larva stained with MitoRos and ConA. Scale bar represents 20 microns.

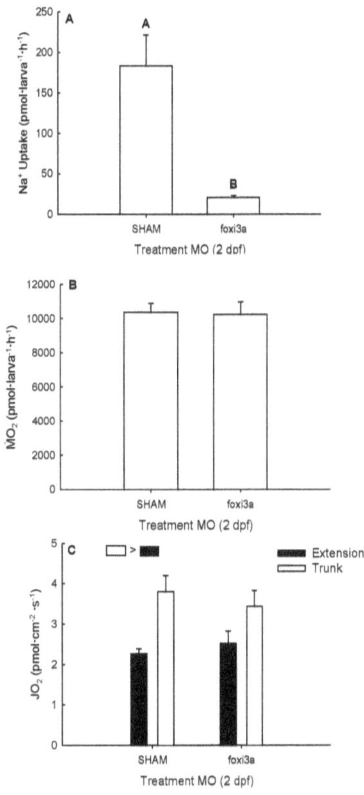

Figure 3.6. The effect of *foxi3a* knockdown on (A) Na^+ uptake, (B) whole-body $\dot{M}O_2$, and (C) epithelial O_2 flux (JO_2) in 2 dpf zebrafish. Larvae were reared and assayed under N-Na and pH 7.6. Differing letters denote a significant different between sham and foxi3a treatments as analyzed using a Student's t-test for Na^+ uptake (MO injection; $p = 0.001$; $n = 8$) and $\dot{M}O_2$ ($p = 0.880$; $n = 11$-15) are denoted by asterisks. There was a significant effect of region on JO_2, denoted by legend in upper left corner of panel C, as determined by a two-way ANOVA followed by a Holm-Sidak post-hoc test (MO injection: $p = 0.861$; region: $p = 0.001$; interaction: $p = 0.343$; $n = 6$).

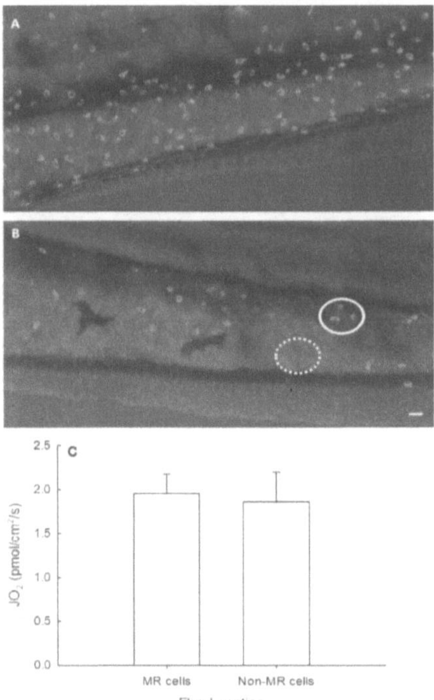

Figure 3.7. A representative image of ionocyte density (along the yolk sac extension of a (A) 3 dpf (A) sham larva is presented along with the decreased ionocyte density of a (B) 3 dpf foxi3a morphant larva. (C) Regional oxygen flux within areas where ionocytes are present and absent along the yolk sac of foxi3a MO-injected larval zebrafish. At 24 hpf, ionocyte density was significantly reduced following the knockdown of foxi3a transcription factor. At 59 hpf, ionocyte density began to return leaving small patches of MitoRos-positive cells (solid line circle in panel B) as well as regions without positive cell staining (dashed line circle in panel B) which could accommodate the tip of the SMOT probe. Larvae were reared under N-Na and pH 7.6. Results were analyzed using a Student's t-test (effect of cell-type: $p = 0.823$. $n = 5$). Scale bar represents 20 microns.

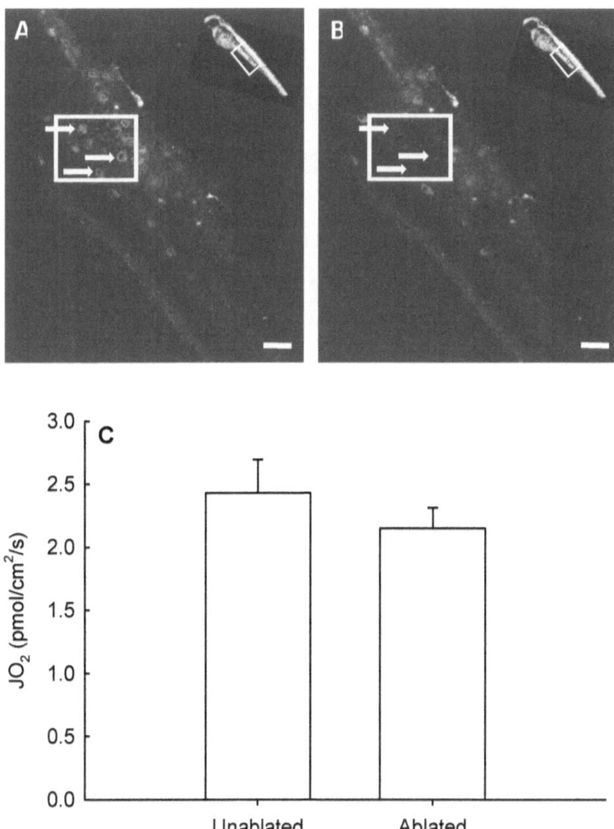

Figure 3.8. Images (A) before and (B) after laser cell ablation highlighting the loss of MitoRos cell stain intensity following ablation are shown. Arrows point to MR cells and the box encircles the target ablation area. Images were enhanced to better visualize ablation. (C) The effect of laser cell ablation on regional JO_2 measured across ablated and unablated regions of the yolk sac extension of 4 dpf larval zebrafish using SMOT. No significant differences were found for JO_2 across the yolk sac extension using a Student's t-test (effect of ablation = 0.387. n = 8). Scale bar represents 20 microns

Chapter 4

General Discussion

For organisms relying on an aerobic metabolism, a constant O_2 supply must be available to energy demanding tissues. Under situations such as low O_2 availability or increased metabolic demands, pressure is placed on the O_2 uptake system of the organism. In this book. the effects of hypoxia exposure and altered ionoregulatory demands on O_2 uptake of the larval zebrafish were evaluated.

4.1 Using micro-optrodes to study aerobic metabolism

Although Chapter 2 and Chapter 3 focus on different areas of fish physiology, a common theme running through this book is the measurement of epithelial JO_2 through SMOT to provide insight into the metabolic demands of underlying tissues and cells. The usage of SMOT is growing within the literature and the applicability of the technique is only beginning to be realized. Micro-optrodes were first applied in aquatic biology to measure O_2 gradients in marine sediments and biofilms (Klimant et al., 1995). Since that study, SMOT has been used in toxicological studies (Sanchez et al., 2008; Stensberg et al., 2014) and has blossomed in the literature of plant physiology to provide estimates of O_2 consumption in plant roots and viability of plant seeds (Ast et al., 2012; Chaturvedi et al., 2013; McLamore et al., 2017). Three papers from the Perry lab (Hughes et al., 2019; Parker et al. 2020; Zimmer et al., 2020), have brought SMOT into the comparative physiology literature. The publication of numerous methods papers (McLamore et al., 2010; McLamore et al., 2017; Porterfield et al., 2006) with the most notable being the comprehensive work of Ferreira et al. (2020) are likely to expand SMOT into even more areas. This book further develops SMOT by using a combinatorial approach employing whole-body O_2 consumption measurements and small-scale JO_2 measures to provide a more holistic view of organismal metabolism.

4.2 A critique of methods

SMOT is still a relatively novel technique and thus it is important to discuss its advantages and limitations. First, the capacity to compartmentalize the O_2 uptake of an organism can address physiological questions that could not be resolved through whole-body respirometry. For example, the decreasing anterior-to-posterior trend of JO_2 which was observed across the larval zebrafish in Chapters 2 and 3 would have been missed by whole-body measurements. Although it might have been possible to detect this trend using O_2 microelectrodes, the sensitivity of this approach has been critiqued with the advent of SMOT (Porterfield et al. 2009). Moreover, some studies have attempted to compartmentalize the body of organisms using a rubber dam method (Rombough, 1998; Wells and Pinder, 1996), however, this technique introduces stress to the animal (as does SMOT) and most importantly cannot be used with smaller organisms such as larval zebrafish. The measurement of O_2 uptake by clusters of ionocytes (Chapter 3) is another example of an advantage of SMOT. With SMOT, we can gain a more direct understanding of near-cellular metabolism as the technique is influenced less by the O_2 consumption of other cell-types and organs. For example, in Chapter 3, after rearing larvae in acidic water, Na^+ uptake increased but JO_2 remained unchanged while whole-body $\dot{M}O_2$ decreased. This discrepancy suggests that other metabolically active tissues are masking and potentially distorting any conclusions relating to the metabolic activity of ionocytes. Indeed, if ion transport costs were more significant than they were determined to be in Chapter 3, it is conceivable that the increased O_2 consumption of the ionocytes might have gone undetected if solely whole-body respirometry had been used.

Admittedly, the real advantage shows itself through the combination of SMOT with whole-body respirometry. Together, they provide the possibility of comparing the same measurements but through different methods to arrive at a more comprehensive and convincing conclusion. For example, larvae must be anesthetized during SMOT which undoubtedly, affects cellular metabolism, however, anesthetic is not needed during whole-body respirometry. It can be imagined that results where JO_2 and $\dot{M}O_2$ concur appear much more convincing than if the results from only one of the techniques were obtained and left to interpret on their own. In cases when the results from both techniques disagree, it provides one with the possibility of discerning impacts that appear negligible at the whole-body level but are more significant when O_2 uptake is considered at a regional level.

At the conception of this book, it was hoped to taper the SMOT tip to a diameter of about 10 microns (40 microns was used in Chapters 2 and 3) to allow measurements from single cells. Although it was physically possible to obtain probes that were 10 microns, the signal-to-noise ratio was too low to provide consistent and reliable measurements (see Supplementary information). Indeed, it is possible miniaturize the SMOT probe even below 10 microns (Porterfield et al. 2010) and still obtain reliable data, however, a laser puller with customized attachments is required to ensure that the fibre is tapered in a way which does not impede or weaken the light transmission properties of the cable.

4.3 Unanswered questions and future directions

In Chapter 2, 4 and 7 dpf larvae were studied. It would be interesting to add other developmental time points to determine how O_2 uptake and vascularization change over time. Moreover, questions such as, "how does hypoxia tolerance change with age?" and, "how does the loss of Hif-1α affect development" could be addressed. It could be hypothesized that the overall spatial pattern of cutaneous JO_2 is likely to change as the gills takes over the role as the primary gas exchanger from the cutaneous surface. Additionally, it could be possible to prevent gill formation through the knockdown of transcription factor *gcm2* (Kwong and Perry, 2015) and observe whether cutaneous O_2 uptake compensates for the loss of gas exchange through the gills. Perhaps by studying different stages, a better understanding of the organ development could be obtained by tracking the major O_2 sinks of the developing zebrafish. Based on the 4 and 7 dpf O_2 map, the highest JO_2 was recorded around the heart and gills. Does this suggest that at this age, these organs are the primary metabolic consumers? Altogether, a potential future study would be to map the changes to O_2 uptake throughout the life cycle of the zebrafish. SMOT could even be used on adult zebrafish to test whether cutaneous gas exchange still contributes to overall O_2 uptake. Using SMOT on larger targets would allow the possibility for intravascular PO_2 measurements. These measurements would be helpful in describing the O_2 transfer across the epithelium as it accounts for the diffusion of O_2 through the epithelium and into the vasculature. In addition, measuring cutaneous thickness would provide a key piece for understanding the diffusion of O_2 across the skin as a thicker epithelium would slow down the rate of diffusion. Notably, JO_2 was found to be different between the middle and the posterior regions at 4 dpf but not at 7 dpf (Figs. 2.2B and 2.5B). This effect may be due to a thickening of the epithelium across the anterior and the middle regions of the older, 7 dpf zebrafish which would explain the lower magnitude of JO_2 measured in these regions. Furthermore, it could also be possible to inject recently developed O_2-sensing microbeads (Robertson, 2017) into the vasculature of the zebrafish to provide real-time visualization of internal PO_2. Finally, SMOT could also be applied in other species. Most notably, air-breathing fish or amphibians since these animals utilize the cutaneous surface for O_2 uptake.

In Chapter 3 the ionoregulatory cost incurred by a larval stage fish was measured, however, a potential future study could be to use SMOT to study the ionoregulatory costs of an adult zebrafish. It would be noteworthy to test whether costs are the same for a larva and an adult, when growth comprises a lesser portion of metabolism and there is a wider aerobic scope. In addition, it would provide data that can easily be compared with other studies in the literature, which have primarily estimated ionoregulatory costs of adult fish. Indeed, the ionocytes of the adult fish are found on the gills rather than the skin, therefore, manipulations will be required to allow the SMOT probe to access these cells. Finally, although challenging, it is suggested that future studies tackling ion transport and SMOT incorporate the scanning ion-selective electrode technique (SIET). It may be possible to run SMOT and SIET simultaneously, which would allow measurements of JO_2 as well as flux rates of specific ions at the same site of measurement. Due to limitations of our SMOT set-up, the incorporation of SIET was not possible.

4.4 Summary and significance

This book broadens our understanding of epithelial O_2 movement, a process that is essential for animals sustaining an aerobic metabolism using cutaneous O_2 uptake. The goal of Chapter 2 was to characterize the epithelium of the larval zebrafish as a gas exchange organ under normoxia and hypoxia and second, to evaluate the role of Hif-1α in managing larval cutaneous O_2 uptake. Regional maps of JO_2 were used to convey the different magnitudes of JO_2 across the body of a larval zebrafish. After hypoxia pre-exposure and the knockout of Hif-1α, the major regulator of maintaining O_2 homeostasis, cutaneous JO_2 remained unchanged. This result did not support the initial hypothesis that was based on the premise that hypoxia-induced compensatory mechanisms regulated by Hif-1a would affect cutaneous JO_2. Nonetheless, the map provides insight into the topography of epithelial O_2 of the larval zebrafish and a detailed understanding of the respiratory physiology of the larval fish. More work remains to be done before a complete understanding of the role of Hif-1α regarding cutaneous O_2 uptake can be achieved.

In Chapter 3, the aerobic cost of ion transport in larval zebrafish was assessed by utilizing SMOT to make near-cellular measurements of JO_2. It was hypothesized that changes in rates of Na^+ uptake evoked by acidic or low Na^+ rearing conditions would result in corresponding changes in whole-body oxygen consumption ($\dot{M}O_2$) and/or JO_2 measured around ionocytes. Larvae that were reared under low pH (pH 4) exhibited a significantly higher rate of Na^+ uptake compared to fish reared under control conditions (pH 7.6) yet displayed a lower $\dot{M}O_2$ and no difference in cutaneous JO_2. Moreover, despite a higher Na^+ uptake capacity in larvae that were reared under low Na^+ conditions, there were no differences in $\dot{M}O_2$ and JO_2. Furthermore, although Na^+ uptake was nearly abolished in 2 dpf larvae lacking ionocytes, $\dot{M}O_2$ and JO_2 were unaffected. Finally, laser ablation of ionocytes did not affect cutaneous JO_2. Thus, it was concluded that the aerobic costs of ion uptake by ionocytes in larval zebrafish, at least in the case of Na^+, are below detection using whole-body respirometry or cutaneous SMOT scans, providing evidence that ion regulation in zebrafish larvae incurs a low aerobic cost. The results of these experiments provide support for the studies in the literature, which have also concluded that ionoregulation in fish is not costly. To date, this is the first study that has addresses the aerobic metabolic costs of ion regulation in a larval-stage fish.

4.5 Concluding remarks

The results of this book display how the measurement of epithelial JO_2 through SMOT can provide significant insight into metabolism. The spatial profiling of JO_2 has revealed that O_2 uptake varies substantially across the epithelium of a cutaneous-respiring larva. The impact of hypoxia-exposure and hif1a knockout was shown to have no effect on the spatial profile of JO_2 across 4 and 7 dpf zebrafish, however, more work remains to understand how this relationship may change through development. Additionally, this book has provided evidence in support of a low aerobic cost associated with ionoregulation in larval fish through the unique perspective of JO_2 measurement above clusters of ionocytes. The combinatorial approach of combining SMOT with whole-body respirometry along with either vasculature analysis (Chapter 2) or radioactive Na^+ tracing (Chapter 3) is a powerful approach for understanding of the metabolic allocation of living organisms. The work presented in this book convincingly wrestles with the challenge of studying sub-organismal metabolism. I hope that the representation of SMOT in this book will inspire future researchers to utilize this technologically-advanced technique to tackle previously untouched questions of science.

www.ingramcontent.com/pod-product-compliance
Lightning Source LLC
LaVergne TN
LVHW041503190726
843491LV00008B/2521

9783384232151